Letters Home

Memoirs of one Army Nurse in the Southwest Pacific in World War II

By

Sally Hitchcock Pullman

First published by AuthorHouse 10/12/04

ISBN: 1-4184-6494-5 (e-book)
ISBN: 1-4184-2789-6 (Paperback)

This book is printed on acid free paper.

Illustrations and cover by the author.
Photographs by the author and friends.

First published by Quickprint 1997

Acknowledgments

I have many to thank for helping me produce my "opus," those who read, proofread, typed, edited and encouraged. Without them, this opus would not have been born.

Big thanks to my daughter Sally, her husband Pekka and my two sons John and David, all of whom pushed me to record these memories and not to stop.

To my five grandchildren without whose constant pressure to write all my stories down I might have given up long ago.

To Dot Lockwood who, over a period of months, urged me to give a program at church about my experiences. This presentation reawakened my memories.

To two friends, Louise Mason and Elizabeth Yoell, who read my 300-page, handwritten manuscript and urged me to publish.

Thanks go to Victor E. Libert, my copyright attorney who, from the goodness of his heart, secured copyright releases for my quotes and secured my original registry with the Library of Congress.

To Bantam Doubleday Dell Publishing Group, Inc., for their kind permission to reprint the paragraph from the book "Immortal Wife" by Irving Stone.

Special thanks to Jakki Garlans who labored long and hard to transcribe my handwritten manuscript into typewritten pages, and whose patience and suggestions were more than appreciated.

To Barbara Askew and Jean Potetz for their help in the preparation of this manuscript.

And to Christie Levandowski for her helpful suggestions and for using her desktop publishing skills to organize the original manuscript into its present format.

Dedication

To all nurses who served anywhere in WWII.

To all my family, my husband, my brother, my children, grandchildren and relatives who have urged me, for many years, to edit my letters home.

To all the nurses with whom I served, whose support, affection and love made my first job in nursing so unforgettable.

To my parents who saved all my letters so I could eventually record my experiences and whose support was endless.

To those special friends, my close Army nursing buddies, Shirl, BC, Betty, Mickey, the men who ferried us around and gave us courage and friendship, and the patients who inspired us.

To the three doctors on my Women's Ward — two Naval doctors, Commanders Lewis and Besseson, and the Army's Major Heath, who took such good care of me when I was sick.

To our chief nurse at the 126th, Major Hortense E. McKay, whose strict discipline and high standards created an exacting and efficient health delivery system which was able and did provide high quality care despite the enormous patient census we carried during the Battle of the Philippines.

To my two sergeants, Bruno and Bannister, whose unswerving and unselfish devotion to duty lightened my very heavy load.

To all the staff of the 126th General who made working there so possible and so pleasant.

To all of those whose love and letters and friendship sustained me during those turbulent months in the Southwest Pacific.

Table of Contents

Acknowledgments v

Dedication vii

Maps xiii

Prologue xvii

Introduction xxi

Becoming a Soldier 1

    Settling In 1

    Basic Training 4

Overseas Assignment 15

    At Sea, *Willard A. Holbrook* USAT.............................. 21

Hollandia, New Guinea 33

    First Impressions.. 33

    Staging — Hollandia 40

    Move to Tent City.. 48

    Detached Service 54th General Hospital 69

    Detached Service 51st General Hospital........................ 71

At Sea, the *Emily H. M. Weder* 89

The Philippines 93

    Leyte.. 95

    January through March... 99

    Detached Service 133rd General Hospital.................... 105

    The 126th General Hospital Opens 109

    History of the 126th General 109

First Head Nurse Assignment — Ward #16 115

Second Head Nurse Assignment Women's Ward #25 121

Nurses from Santo Tomas.. 123

April through June.. 135

Adventure to Carigara 135

Amoeba 144

Trip to the *Admiral Hershey* *165*

Nurse — Surgery, Ward #6 168

Head Nurse — Dermatology, Ward #4 183

Trip to the Old Fort.. 184

July through September 187

Transfer to Orthopedics, Ward #24... 187

Promotion to 1st Lieutenant... 190

The War is Over.. 196

Accolades to the 126th General.. 203

The 77th Division Dance at Cebu 207

We move to the 73rd Field Hospital Army of Occupation 210

Detached Service 116th Station Hospital....................................... 211

October through November 213

Detached Service 44th General Hospital 218

Relieved of Duty — Replacement Depot.. 221

Going Home... **225**

At Sea on the *Harry Lee*, Navy APA... 225

Delay in Honolulu 226

Stateside — San Diego to Fort Dix 229

A Private Car and the Trip Home... 229

Fort Dix, New Jersey..233

Home 233

Epilogue **237**

Maps

Pacific Theater..24

Southwest Pacific Area 1944 30

New Guinea and Surrounding Islands 1944............................30

Enlarged Map of Dutch New Guinea 1944 31

The Philippine Archipelago...91

Main Islands in My Text 1945..92

Leyte Island – Locations of Familiar Places 1945 171

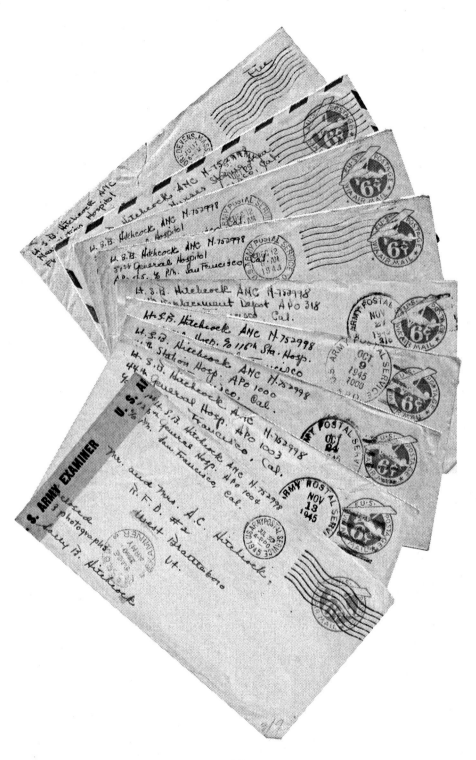

xv

Prologue

As I sat in the glassed-in cocktail lounge, called The Top of the Mark at the top of the Mark Hopkins Hotel in San Francisco on February 12, 1997, I was painfully nostalgic. To look out over the twinkling lights in the harbor, to see the graceful spans of lights on the bridges, and the beauty of the city lights just coming on below, was lovely. It was made more beautiful by the sun setting behind the mountains, at the edge of our country. All gave me a feeling of joy it is hard to express.

Music was flowing endlessly from the fingers of a talented pianist who used no music. He was sitting at a grand piano playing old songs, new ones, and classical ones. What a background for many of my memories.

My daughter Sal and I each sipped a glass of wine as we listened and waited for Sal's husband to join us. Both of us were enjoying the music and the breathtaking view.

It was the music that did it for me! I was compelled to go up to the musician with my $5.00 to tell him how much we were enjoying his playing.

He smiled, "Do you have a favorite song?" he asked.

"I love 'Laura'," I replied.

"A-ha, an oldie from World War II," he responded, smiling.

"Yes," I answered, "Fifty-three years ago, I passed San Francisco in a troop ship bound for the Pacific Theater. I was an Army Nurse. That ship was as close as I've ever been to this city until today! On the way across the Pacific we used to hear endlessly about The Top of the Mark. I have always wanted to come. Now I'm finally here! Thank you so much for your concert."

For a large part of the following hour, my "friend" played WWII songs. The melodies I loved washed over the room and Sal and me. Each time he'd play an old song, he'd give us a "thumbs up" and a big smile.

My whole experience in the service seemed to well up and come alive again in my memory as I remembered New Guinea and the Philippines, all the joys, the sadness, fears, frustrations, sickness and health, courage and pain. It was my first professional job as a nurse for I had just graduated from Yale University School of Nursing with a Masters in Nursing. It was the biggest challenge of my life.

That evening, I decided to edit the boxes of letters I had written home to my parents and to friends who were kind enough to save my letters to them. So fifty-three years later, grounded by a broken leg, I have compiled this story. It is how I saw it, felt it, lived it and expressed it to loved ones and friends at home.

I have interrupted my story occasionally with excerpts from Army papers and with descriptions of areas needing an explanation. The majority of this story is an exact copy of my words from another place, from another time. Best of all are the vivid and long-lasting memories that seem to be with me still—memories of the wonderful friends and associates whose lives intermeshed with mine during those intense months. I will never forget the richness that real friendship brings. That richness and warmth lasts a lifetime.

Introduction

June 1944 was a very tense time for the world and for my family. D-Day, June 6, 1944, had finally happened. Our troops had gone ashore in Normandy for the long- awaited invasion of mainland Europe. My brother John was a Navy pilot flying shore patrols in PB4Ys (Army B-24s) on antisubmarine duty out of England. We worried about him constantly, especially because we had had no news from him in many days.

I, his younger sister, had graduated from Smith College three years before, with a major in geology and a minor in history. Thirty-six months later, I was newly graduated from Yale with a Masters Degree in Nursing. I had passed my physical exam for the Army Nurse Corps in the spring just before graduation.

In early June, I traveled to my parent's home in Brattleboro, Vermont. They had moved to Vermont from Bristol, Connecticut in 1943 at my Dad's retirement. I had grown up and been educated in

Bristol and had gone from there to college and nurses' training. Now Vermont was home and I arrived there with my graduate degree and my State of Connecticut nursing license in hand and began the wait for my orders. There were wars on two fronts, one in Europe, now in full swing, and the other in the Pacific where slowly, General Douglas MacArthur was beginning to retake the huge area under Japanese control.

In this tense time, I waited to be called to active duty. Despite my mother's horror at my wanting to serve, I felt compelled to go to help. My orders finally came.

I remember my Dad coming in with the mail on June 13, 1944 and saying, "Lieutenant, your papers have come!" My heart began to pound. There was a long, neat, white envelope. I remember sitting in the living room on that sunny day unfolding my papers.

"I have to be sworn in!" I said, stupidly.

Dad grinned, "Come on, let's go to the Postmaster."

Off we went to the Postmaster, and I was duly sworn in as a Second Lieutenant in the Army Nurse Corps. Mom and Dad were proud. I was so excited. When I arrived home, there in the window next to my brother's was another Service Star — a six-inch by six-inch white tile with a red inch-wide border and a blue star in the white center. This was for me! I was touched.

Next day another formidable envelope arrived. It was very heavy. I opened it. On the top was printed, "RESTRICTED" in red ink. I looked at the first paragraph and gulped in confusion. I tried again but ended up knowing two things. I was to report for active duty to Fort Devens in Ayer, Massachusetts on June 21, 1944, as 2nd Lt. Sally B. Hitchcock - ANC, N-752998.

And so it was, on June 21, 1944 I was on my way. My Mom and Dad borrowed gas coupons to drive me from Brattleboro to Greenfield, Massachusetts where I boarded the train to Ayer, Massachusetts, the site of Fort Devens.

This was a highly significant time in my life. I was going to my very first job as a graduate nurse. I was 25 years old and had been in school for the past 19 years of my life. I was excited and determined to use all my training to help mend as many injured men and women as I could, and help them come home to their families and loved ones. So many of my friends were serving. It was a personal goal and a promise!

As I sat in that old railroad car (WWI vintage), with its green plush seats and no air conditioning, I was terribly aware of how hard this leave-taking was for my Mom and Dad. My brother John was somewhere in Europe. I was going to be somewhere else. Neither of my parents was young anymore.

The train puffed along and I kept saying to myself, in time to the clicking rails, "I want to go, I want to go." Whether I sat next to anyone else I can't recall, but I remember I tried to read "Taps for Private Tussie."[1]

---

[1] A popular novel in 1944.

I blotted my damp hands. I looked out at the bright, cloudless June day at the cozy farms and small homes neatly placed in their space and I said to myself "Calm down, you sissy. Read your book and relax!"

A soldier walked down the aisle for water. "Should I ask him how far Ayer is?"

"Sit tight," I said to myself, "You'll find out soon enough!"

"Ayer and Fort Devens!" the conductor called as his head appeared for a moment at the front door of the car. That was my stop!

Slowly, I got my bag and pocketbook and stepped off. Now where? I looked around and saw nothing there. A sign with a single word caught my eye — "INFORMATION." What a wonderfully warm word that was. I went over and asked the woman how to get to Fort Devens. "Which department?" she asked. I wasn't sure. She suggested I take a taxi.

No taxis—I stood waiting. On the platform, a sergeant was lining men up for a bus. "There's where I should be," I thought," behind those new Army recruits." A man came up to me from his parked station wagon. He was a sergeant with the nicest face, graying hair and he said with a smile, "You look lost. May I help you?" The station wagon said Fort Devens, USA. I told him my quandary and he laughed.

"Come with me, Lieutenant, I'm going right up there." Such relief I've never known. We drove off and with a smile and a flourish of orders we sailed through gates and up to the location on my orders.

"You wait here, I'll sign you in and get you to your quarters." I waited in the car. Out he came and drove me to a barracks where he unloaded my bag and told me my room number. He saluted and drove off.

I can't remember his name and I wish I could! We had mutual friends and we had fun talking. How I wish I could have told him in words how grateful I was. He knew though, I'm sure, for he'd seen my plight on the platform and he'd known my confusion.

Here I was. I found my room. It was dark inside and hot. My quarters were in one of the buff-colored, wooden, one-storied buildings that spread in Army precision over acres of sandy soil. "Leftovers from WWI," I thought. There were hundreds, all the same but each was numbered. That helped.

My room was unadorned. I had a bed, bureau, a chair and a closet. How hot it was. No air conditioning here. The walls were covered with brown building paper. There were water stains on the ceiling.

I was here. It was my goal! Suddenly there was a knock on my door. There were four of my Yale classmates, Selma, Anne, Shirley and Mildred! It was good to see them. Mildred, who had arrived a month before, was to be our guide.

Chapter One

Becoming a Soldier

Settling In

At this date, Army nurses had only "relative rank." Our uniforms were not the same as regular Army. We wore white uniforms, white caps, white stockings and shoes. Our sweater was Navy blue, as was the lovely, heavy cape with the maroon lining. We received our nurses' insignia ANC, our gold second lieutenant bars and our dog tags on chains. Also issued to us were sheets, blankets, towels, washcloths, and a mattress cover we learned could be used as a shroud.

New Station Hospital, Fort Devens, Massachusetts

June 25, 1944

Dear Mom and Dad,

I can't believe I'm sitting here in our attractive sitting room with a rug like the one in our living room and a lamp like the one in the library. Already I've worked on the wards, brand new graduate that I am. I learned so much. All that is missing is a pair of GI water wings! Not a dry day so far.

The day after I arrived, we had our physical exams. I was fitted with a pair of GI glasses with metals rims. Then we were outfitted with two pairs brown walking shoes, two pairs white nursing shoes, one overseas coat, one rain coat, two ties, ten insignia, one pair high training shoes, two suit coats (size 10) for winter, two suit skirts (size 14 short), one blue cape, one dress hat, three uniforms (white), six white nursing hats, two pairs gloves (one leather, one wool) and two fatigue shirts.

What a wardrobe! It was for winter so Shirl, Selma and I went into Ayer to buy two fatigue dresses which are lightweight and cost $18.00. One is olive drab, the other beige and maroon. We bought two overseas hats. I walked into a size 11 with no alterations. What a shock!

The ward where I have been assigned is an upper respiratory ward. It is good to be working — I do enjoy nursing so much. We only have 10 patients and I gave two baths and made up the rest of the beds. I was in charge. The guys do appreciate a kindly grin. One said when I woke him today, "Oh, boy! This is my idea of heaven. What a morale builder! My first stop after the war will be in Vermont!"

The rain goes on. Seems like it's rained every day since we got here and some of the nurses' rooms leak. Mine was dry, but so many rooms were wet that we were all moved to another barracks.

The food is wonderful — green vegetables, fresh fruit, salads, and all the milk you want. German POWs wait on the table. They are so very young and they work very hard. We can't talk to them or acknowledge their presence. I wonder what they think of America and its Army and us. Armed MPs stand along the edge of the dining area.

Went to the movies last night for 15¢. On the way over, a 1st lieutenant laughed at us and said, "Uniform coats must be buttoned at all times!" Ours were wide open letting in the cool air. Oh, my! Army rules!!

Tomorrow we start Basic Training for four weeks — two weeks of drill and classes and two weeks on the wards. Then we have another graduation and another diploma. I thought I'd had my last in April, but I guess not. I'm at it again.

Love, Sally B.[2]

I recall —

Sometime during the first two or three weeks, we nurses were informed that we had gained "full status!" No more "relative rank." We had to replace our first issue of clothes. The white uniforms, hats, stockings, shoes and blue sweater and cape all became excess baggage and I sent everything home.

In place of these items, our uniforms became brown and white seersucker wraparounds and a strange seersucker "stove pipe" cap.

---

[2] "Sally B." was my family's name for me. The "B" being for my middle name — Bradley.

Dress uniforms, visor caps, overseas capes, coats, skirts, cotton and woolen blouses with ties, fatigues, brown high shoes, wool socks, olive drab raincoat, an olive drab cape, sweater, wool scarf and slacks became our wardrobe. Basic was in full tilt.

Basic Training

For a month, we went to classes to learn Army nursing, discipline, rules, courtesy. We learned about poison gasses and gas raids. Every hour from 6 a.m. to 6 p.m. was filled with learning.

Each morning our casual group (new inductees) had an hour of calisthenics with WAC 1st Lt. Fagan. She was a beautiful woman — straight, thin, tall, muscular, with curly short dark hair, snapping black eyes and she was a "slave driver!" We did exercises. We did push-ups. We marched in every direction until it was a perfect thing.

Each day before it got too hot we "built muscle." The reason was soon apparent! At the end of four weeks of Basic we were to have a day in the field to be "tested." It was a scorching hot Saturday in mid-July in sandy Ayer.

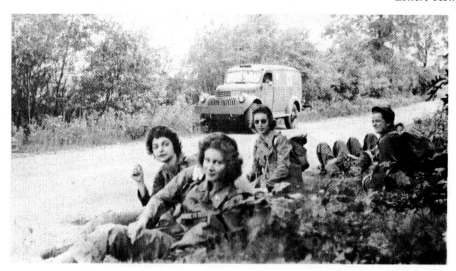

Selma, Shirl, Anne and Edna on rest during the famous basic hike with an ambulance in the background.

We donned our fatigues, back packs, canteens, gas masks, helmets, high shoes with wool socks and set off. We had a good packful of equipment we'd need, so with our gear loaded, we began the march. It seemed like ten miles. Our fatigues were new and very stiff. It was hot and nothing "breathed." An ambulance followed us just in case someone was unable to continue. One gal had trouble so she went into the ambulance.

Finally, we arrived at a large open field where we were told to relax and prepare for lunch. We were glad to sit down and eat and drink.

Many important "big brass" were there — majors from the ANC HQ (Army Nurse Corps Headquarters) in Boston, our own major from Fort Devens, others of higher rank, both men and women.

Fagan's training was on display. We marched "forward, reverse, right turn, left turn, right oblique, left oblique" all to her clear commands. Suddenly, I discovered that the nurse I'd always *followed* in line had been picked up in the ambulance. So there I was leading off one line and I had never done well with my "right" and "left."

The rapid commands came, then a "left oblique;" my line was two people ahead of the lines on either side and I went *"right."* I found myself all alone and wrong! I was sure I'd be reprimanded or discharged! That was problem number one.

The second problem was the tear gas test. We were protected from the tear gas bombs they threw at us by our masks. But I had a bee in my mask! I frantically ran to the side, pulled off my mask, shooed the bee away while holding my breath and then pulled the mask on again. I ran back to the group.

I was questioned. All of the brass must have thought about the wisdom of continuing the relationship between the Nurse Corps and me. But I graduated after four weeks from Basic Training. Another graduation!

July 9, 1944

Dear Mom and Dad,

We've had drill and class each day and yesterday we had final exams. I got 100 in Military Courtesy; however, in the other exams I didn't do quite so well.

Social life is active this week. The officers' club had an outdoor clambake. My first. There was a huge pile of hot rocks covered with seaweed and then clams and lobsters. A canvas was pulled over everything. For a New Englander, this was my first experience with a clambake. It was delicious. The Army tries so hard to keep us happy!

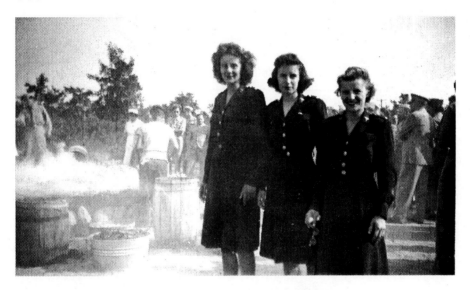

Shirl, Anne and me at the Fort Devens clambake.

I'm working on two isolation floors. Quite different technique from Yale! So many guys on this floor were sent home with malaria. They are so sick when the chills hit and we have to give ice water sponges, have a fan blowing on them trying to get the spiking temperatures down. The fevers are so high! It is a brand new experience.

There are other strange problems on this floor, diseases I have to look up — tropical diseases like schistosomiasis, dengue and amoebic dysentery.

(*I should have seen the handwriting on the wall, but did not.*)

Love, Me

July 23, 1944

Dear Folks,

After graduation, I was assigned to night duty (7 p.m. – 7 a.m.) at the hospital called Lovell South. The ward I'm on is plastic surgery and skin diseases. There is a wonderful group of patients here and I'm getting along well. My charge nurse is fine! I'm called "Miss Hitch"! Much amusement over my name. Sometimes Hiscok, Hotchkiss, Wild Bill Hickox. Hitchcock comes hard! Now I'm to go on nights.

Our chief nurse is remarkable, the youngest major. I'm glad to be here at Lovell. My room is nicer, a comfortable bed, bureau, lamps and a desk with a chair. The walls are thicker so that the rooms are cooler. Shirl and I are in the same barracks. It's nice she's here. We both miss Anne who was separated from us to fill another nurse's place to go to Hawaii when the first nurse flunked her physical. Anne was a wonderful sport! "Stiff upper lip and all that." We hated to have her go.

Yes, I'm truly glad to be here. I love my nursing. I'm so glad I have this wonderful training with which I can do so much good. Now I'm in charge of four wards at night with two ward men on each ward. Somehow I managed to get done the first night and now each night is easier.

One of my ward men is Don Glew who wanted to be in medical school but now helps me as a corpsman. He is funny, able and artistic. Here are some of his drawings.

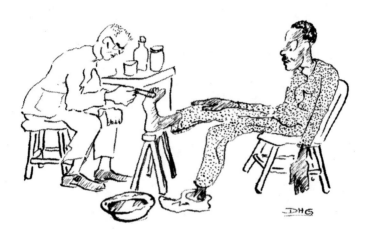

Original drawings, on this and the following page, were given to me by Don Glew at Fort Devens

Trying to sleep days is another problem. The nickelodeon is in the day room next to my quarters. Records play all day — Andrews Sisters, the Ink Spots, Benny Goodman, Glen Miller, Tommy Dorsey, and "Der Bingo" — all the special ones, hour-after-hour. Eventually I sleep, but not well.

Love, Sally B.

I remember —

Back to nights and my many dressings. I will never forget one episode. It was the skin and plastic surgery ward. Don and I had been doing endless soaks and dressings between 7 and 9 p.m.

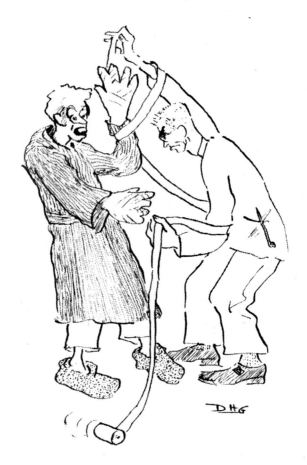

One night a big uncomplaining patient, who had dressings on both legs from his groin to his feet, hobbled up to us asking for a sleeping pill because he was so uncomfortable. I checked his orders and then gave him a Nembutal.

Don and I watched him as he stiffly padded to his bed halfway down the ward. We both saw him hesitate and then fall to his knees beside his bed, head down. We rushed after him and spoke to him.

"Jones, Jones, what is it? Are you all right?"

No response.

Pulse normal.

Don shook him gently. No response.

"What is it, Jones? Are you dizzy?" I asked.

A bass voice from deep within said, "Gee, Mam, can't a man even say his prayers?" Life was many things, but never dull.

While I was on nights, Shirl came bursting into my room. "Wake up, we're assigned!"

"Where?" I gasped.

"The Southwest Pacific!" she responded.

"When?"

"Next week!"

Somewhere in Basic, we'd been asked to sign-up for our choice of theaters in which to serve. Of course, we all signed up for Europe. Since D-Day, June 6, 1944, Europe was in the full throes of the invasion. But we were all assigned to go to the Pacific where MacArthur, by island hopping, by terrible invasions and human loss, was slowly, inexorably recapturing the enormous Pacific area taken over in 1941-42 by the Japanese.

These were frantic days of getting clothes issue, stamping clothes, labeling footlockers and suitcases, getting all the right papers, clearing the post, making wills, getting shots and writing letters.

August 15, 1944

Dear Mom and Dad,

Another night has gone and a busy one at that. It's been so busy with all these wards. Days are so hot; I don't sleep well so I haven't written regularly.

A big surprise came this past week. I'm being transferred. Where, I don't know, but don't worry if you don't hear for a bit. I'll let you know as soon as I can where I am. Shirley and I are together. I'm glad of that.

I hate to leave. I've loved working here. I admire the nursing staff. I enjoy my work and my patients. It comes over me in waves how much I owe you both for my education. What a rich and wonderful one and now it is bringing real returns in service and personal satisfaction.

Just a note on my first night duty. I have enjoyed it even though 12 hours is a long haul. Some of the patients call me "Mom"! Am I that maternal? It's been a lot of fun! How glad I am I chose nursing as a profession!

Love, Sally B.

I recall —

On August 15, 1944, we were assigned to a group of 33 New England nurses, many just out of school. We were under the leadership of 1st Lts. Loretta Shultz and Dorothy Huse who remained our senior officers all the way west and beyond. Every one of those women was a friend. With the exception of two, we stayed together to the end.

RESTRICTED
Army Service Forces
Headquarters First Service Command
Boston 15, Massachusetts

17 August 1944

SPECIAL ORDERS
NO. 230

Extracts

*   *   *

1. The following named nurses, ANC, are relieved from further assignment and duty at FSC Basic Training Center for ANC, SCU 3115, Fort Devens, Massachusetts, and WP to Camp Stoneman, Pittsburg, California, to as to arrive on 25 August 1944, reporting upon arrival to CO for disposition:

```
1ST LT LAURETTA SLATE SCHULZ, N-721890, MOS 3430 (LTD SERV)
1ST LT DOROTHY HUSE, N-752144, MOS 3430
2D LT PHYLLIS M. KENDREW, N-752682, MOS 3437
2D LT BERNICE P. BURNS, N-752986, MOS 3443 (LTD SERV)
2D LT RUTH W. DAILEY, N-752904, MOS 3443 (LTD SERV)
2D LT DOROTHY H. ACKERLY, N-752900, MOS 3449
2D LT MYRTLE E. ARD, N-752967, MOS 3449
2D LT AMIE C. BALLOU, N-752993, MOS 3449
2D LT ALICE M. BARTKIAVICUS, N-752901, MOS 3449
2D LT REBECCA M. BENEDICT, N-752929, MOS 3449
2D LT JUNE B. BICKMORE, N-752968, MOS 3449
2D LT MILDRED DAMON, N-752971, MOS 3449
2D LT IRENE E. DOYLE, N-752919, MOS 3449
2D LT PRISCILLA W. MCWILLIAM, N-752957, MOS 3449
2D LT HELEN M. PAULUCCY, N-752962, MOS 3449
2D LT IRENE J. PIDLOWSKA, N-752947, MOS 3449 (LTD SERV)
2D LT RITA M. PROFENNO, N-752574, MOS 3449
2D LT MARY A. PRONCKO, N-752959, MOS 3449
2D LT BEULAH C. LARSON, N-753000, MOS 3449
2D LT MARY T. FAHEY, N-752975, MOS 3449
2D LT DERNIECE N. GAHAGAN, N-752985, MOS 3449
2D LT EDNA L. LAMBERT, N-752979, MOS 3449 (LTD SERV)
2D LT MARY K. WESOLY, N-752995, MOS 3449
2D LT ELIZABETH F. KNOWLES, N-752978, MOS 3449
2D LT LILLIAN M. MAGUIRE, N-752987, MOS 3449
2D LT VIRGINIA A. JONES, N-753001, MOS 3449
2D LT THELMA F. RAINEY, N-752642, MOS 3449
2D LT HELEN I. ROSLONOWSKI, N-752990, MOS 3449
2D LT SALLY B. HITCHCOCK, N-752998, MOS 3449
2D LT SHIRLEY K. MUNSON, N-752996, MOS 3449
2D LT LUCIA M. TOMPKINS, N-752989, MOS 3449
```

TDN. FDS 501-31 P431-02-03-07-08 212/50425. The TC will furnish the necessary T.

By command of Major General MILES:

W. A. BARRON, JR.
Colonel, General Staff Corps
Chief of Staff

Official

O. L. FARNSWORTH,
Colonel, Adjutant General's Department

RESTRICTED

(over)

NURSES ASSIGNED TO THE PACIFIC THEATER
ORDERS — AUGUST 17, 1944

CHAPTER TWO

Overseas Assignment

I remember —

On August 16, 1944, we left Fort Devens for the West Coast. The train was long and loaded with troops. Thirty-three of us were in a Pullman car designed for 28. Some of us had to double up, so Shirl and I slept head to toe in a lower berth all the way west. We didn't sleep much!

There were wonderful women in this group but five of us formed a special and long-lasting bond, Beulah Christina "BC" Larsen, Elizabeth "Knowlsey" Knowles, Shirley Munson, Lillian "Mickey" McGuire and me. BC, Shirl, and I still write. Knowlsey and Mickey are gone. Such a special bond is a rare and cherished thing.

It was wonderful for me to look out the train windows taking in our huge country — the eastern mountains, the Great Plains, the mountains in the west. I'd been to Yellowstone and Glacier Parks with my family. I'd been to Washington, Idaho, Montana and the Dakotas with friends. I'd spent a summer studying field geology at the University of Wyoming Summer Science School, but never had I been west through Salt Lake and the Sierras to California. That was where we were going.

August 25, 1944

Dear Mom and Dad,

It was a glorious trip to this place on the West Coast. We had a Pullman car to ourselves and Shirley and I bunked together in a lower berth. We rode through Ohio and Indiana to Chicago where we had a layover. Five of us went to the movies then to the Bismarck Hotel for supper. Of course one cup of coffee was 25¢ so we didn't have many! We walked a lot in Chicago seeing the stores and more stores and even the lake.

Late that night we left on our troop train for Iowa. Shirl and I rode miles on the back of the train with the conductor and the trainman who answered our many questions.

We saw the place where the Golden Spike at Council Bluffs was driven. We rushed off to buy a box lunch at the station then back on board to arrive at Omaha. All that day and night we crossed Nebraska. It's so long.

Soon it was Wyoming and Cheyenne where we got out to buy an ice cream cone. How good to be back in the country where I did my field work in geology at the University of Wyoming Summer

Science School. But I slept through Laramie where the University is! Couldn't believe it.

Next day we stopped in Ogden, Utah and saw Great Salt Lake. Clear as could be were the old beach levels of Lake Bonneville, the huge glacial lake of which Salt Lake is a remnant. We looked at this huge salt-water lake seeing patterns of floating salt. The water is bright blue green.

It was incredible to me to be crossing the great salt desert — miles and miles of white salt and sand. I thought of those first pioneers who crossed with little water, behind slow moving beasts. How terribly brave they were! Far to the west were the high mountains which they and now we would cross. How different the circumstances!!

We have some wonderful diversions. One is our porter, Hubert Kelsoe. He is so nice and does anything for us. The other is the conductor on our Pullman, Bill Mooney, who comes into our car every night to sing. He has a marvelous voice and knows every song there is to know. So we all join in and the music flows!

We have arrived here safely (*Camp Stoneman, Pittsburg, California*) on an arm of San Francisco Bay. Everyone is friendly. It is beautiful here with lovely mountains to our east and west. But I'm ready to sleep. It will be good to sleep in a bed alone after four nights with Shirl in that lower berth.

I've washed my hair, clothes, repacked, and treated my sunburned nose. How strange to realize a week ago I was home! Our room looks like a tailor shop, skirts and shirts all over. The bed is the only empty spot. I'm ready! Goodnight for now!

Love, me

I recall —

Camp Stoneman, just east of San Francisco, was a debarkation depot for the Army. We had traveled by train through the brownest valley I'd ever seen. Then we were there.

Our agenda was full. We began classes on "secrecy." We were campused. We were sworn to secrecy. We had to pack our cameras and destroy our diaries. We had more shots: typhus, typhoid, and cholera. We had already had tetanus and smallpox. We were so full of protection, we felt we could drink from the Ganges.

I cannot remember much of Stoneman. I do remember eating my very first tree-ripened orange. It was so sweet!

It was a hectic time having orders checked, getting shots, repacking my suitcase and footlocker, both now stamped with my identification:

Lt. Sally B. Hitchcock ANC, N-752998

Pleasant Valley Road

West Brattelboro, Vermont

We were at Camp Stoneman only 48 hours. The next day we knew we would be moving again. At noon the men began to march under full pack. It was very hot. We were told it was 110°. Somehow our lieutenants had commandeered a truck for us and we rode slowly past platoon after platoon of walking men. We felt for those men as we arrived at the covered dock in Oakland, where we unloaded. There was a huge ship, the *Willard A. Holbrook* USAT (United States Army Transport), formerly the *President Taft*, a huge transoceanic pleasure liner, converted by the Army into a troopship.

Red Cross ladies were handing out donuts and coffee or milk. I drank a lot of milk, knowing it would be a while before I would have any again! The dock was dark. A cheer went up from the ship's rails above, "NURSES!" I'd heard catcalls before, but never so loud or so many! It was a cheery welcome. A band played for hours and still the men came. The dock was jammed.

There was an end to the embarkees. We were assigned to quarters, seven to a first-class stateroom for two. We were also assigned to a seat in the dining room and given a meal ticket. Many Army and Naval officers and flyers were aboard. There were over 3,000 enlisted men quartered in the swimming pools, on the decks, in every possible available space on that ship. We were 33 casuals, plus three returning nurses. The rest were our men.

T. S. Form No. 160a   Formerly Q. M. C. Form No. 160a
(Revised June 19, 1942)

UNITED STATES ARMY TRANSPORT
FIRST CLASS

Name	*Stateroom*
HITCHCOCK, SALLY B. 2ND LT.	117
RM 033 (d)	

Sitting [First / Second] 3   Table No. 2   Seat Nos. _____

(Please present this card to dining room steward at first meal served after sailing.)

16—20052-1

Meal ticket for table #2, 3rd sitting.

As I look back today, I am awed by the logistics of providing food, water, medicine and entertainment for this many people for the 21 days we would be at sea.

Our ship was to sail unescorted to its destination, the first unescorted troop ship to cross the Pacific I was told. I'm not sure this was true.

The night was clear and beautiful. Shirl and I went topside in our lined coats that not so long before we had thought of not packing. There were many Navy men and Navy flyers, as well as Army officers, all topside. They were going as replacements for the Army, Navy, and the Air Corps and for the ships so gamely carrying troops and cutting Japanese supply lines. Theirs was to be an active future!

We all sat on the deck that night looking at the twinkling lights of the cities of Oakland and San Francisco and the tiny moving "fireflies" crossing the Oakland Bridge. I met a young philosopher on deck that night, a flier. We both filled our eyes with the warm sight of home we knew we would not see again for a while. Here we heard a new slogan, "Golden Gate in '48!" We all said it again and again.

At Sea, *Willard A. Holbrook* USAT

At 0900 on August 27, 1944, we set sail! Before anyone was up, Shirl and I got up. Everything was cloaked in dense fog. Quietly, so as not to wake our five roommates, we went topside.

We felt adrift in the fog and in our lives. There was neither end nor any beginning. We were on water we could not see, going somewhere we did not know. Our thoughts turned inward as the fog engulfed us both. We stood a long time peering into our past and wondering about our future, wondering what the other nurses were thinking about, wondering what the fighting men were thinking about. We even spoke of getting home and we had not yet even left.

Would our world be the same? Would our families, our special friends, our loved ones be the same? What were they doing now? Flights of ideas swarmed. We were suddenly cut off from the familiar, the secure, the loving and had joined the many people all facing this big unknown. We both felt it all and said so, "We have to do our best. We have a job to do."

The breakfast bell rang. Shirl and I made a dash for chow. Our first day on board had begun!

No one knew where we were headed. We plowed past Alcatraz and slipped under the Golden Gate Bridge that we could barely see over our heads and sailed out of the homeport of San Francisco. The bridge's giant span loomed through the fog. The ship's foghorn gave a mournful blast every few minutes. It was eerie. Its cry went on day and night, another day and night until we sailed out of the thick blanket of fog which had covered us for so long.

Scuttlebutt began. "Where are we going?" Rumors were rampant. Some swore we'd get off in Hawaii. I hoped so because that's where Anne was. Some said India, others Australia. We had days to play guessing games because as the ship's captain told us, "I can't tell you anything for my orders are sealed!"

In August, the Pacific Ocean is beautiful. There were days when the clouds and sea were unbelievable. In the evening when the sun was setting and the sky became pink, I couldn't tell where the ocean stopped and the sky began. Mists blurred the line of the horizon and the sky. Big as it was, the ocean seemed small, intimate with us in our ship in the center of a small, round world.

Sometimes at night, in the disturbed waters of our bow waves, there was a green glow of phosphorescence. Sometimes we would see flying fish lift out of the water trailing silver drops of water behind. We did see porpoise a few times.

The days were long, but each of us was going to "the duty." In just a few days, one of our pilot friends informed us that Hawaii had been bypassed, that we were heading southwest. We were traveling on the perimeter of the newly-won-back island territories in the Southwest Pacific.

We had long talks with the men and other nurses. Constantly we heard about the Top of the Mark in San Francisco, a cocktail lounge where so many officers had spent time. It was a lovely spot, they said, at the top of the Mark Hopkins Hotel on top of Nob Hill. Everyone who went to Frisco had to go there. It became a symbol of home.

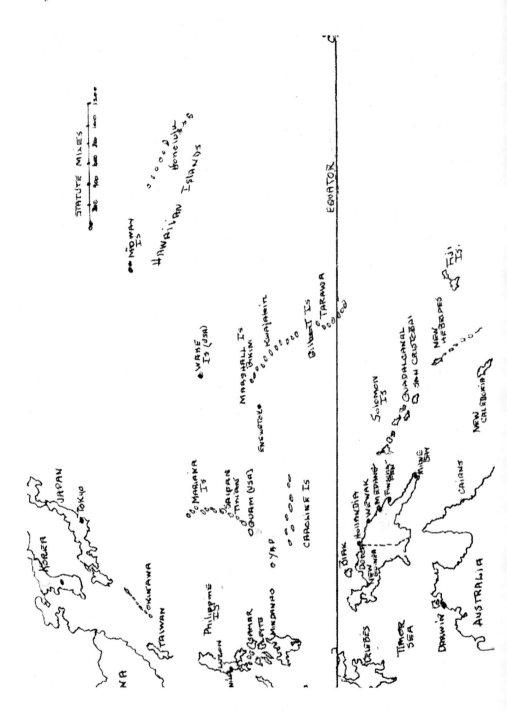

MAP OF THE PACIFIC OCEAN IN 1944

There were foolish shipboard romances, tragic because they were so real and painful. Some men were glad to leave home, some sweating it out to get home — aching for their wives and kids, men who were homesick and others, with a "Let me at 'em attitude," who thought the whole excursion was a lark. They were a real cross-section of our youth.

Almost all of us went to chapel. BC, Shirl and I sang in the ship's choir with other officers and enlisted men. We sang for both the Catholic and Protestant services. It was fun. There were some beautiful voices in that choir.

They were a wonderful bunch of guys and gals! We had fun. We played cards, tag and jumped rope. We just talked.

Frequently we had boat drill. We donned our life jackets and helmets and ran to our assigned stations. We never knew when it might be the real thing. And we never knew what was under us or in front of us as we sped across that huge ocean.

Once we began to zigzag. We speeded up — a big increase in speed. No one was told why. It just was. We were all scared when the boat drill alarm sounded. We donned our life jackets and helmets. We flew to our stations where the word was, "It is a submarine on our port side!" With clammy hands and a fast heartbeat, we waited.

Suddenly a huge mass appeared from the water. We could hardly breathe. It was a whale! What a relief! What a shock! What an enormous animal! We were so lucky. There were no other incidents, but none of us ever forgot that one.

About fifteen days out, we began to take daily atabrine pills. We knew this was malaria prevention. More scuttlebutt—not India, not Australia; it had to be some islands in the Southwest Pacific area.

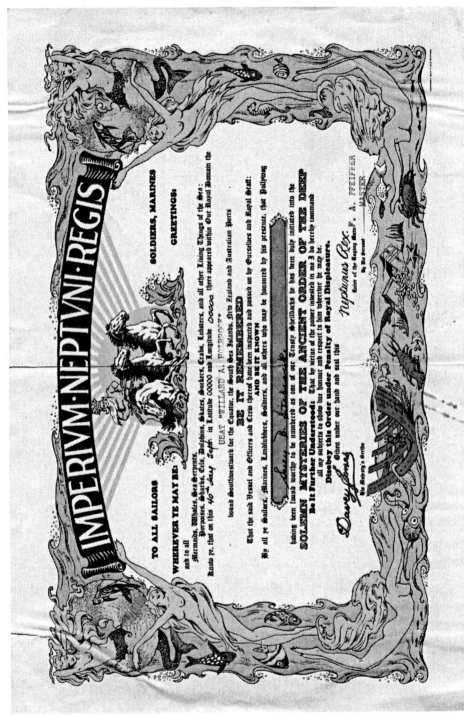

International Dateline Diploma

One of the great fun-things that happened was the day we all became "Shellbacks." When the ship crossed the equator we had a huge "Do" on the ship. Everyone was involved.

There was shaving of heads, beards, dunking, kissing flour, much laughter by everyone and we all got certificates stating that "...on the 40th Day of September in Latitude 0000 and Longitude 0000, there appeared within our Royal Domain the USAT *Willard A. Holbrook* bound southwestward for the Equator, South Sea Islands, New Zealand and Australian Ports. ... And be it known ... that pollywog, (name of person) has been found worthy to be numbered as one of our Trusty Shellbacks ..." We all got certificates!

Occasionally, we began to see volcanic peaks on the horizon. It was land. Each seemed to wear a cloud ring about halfway up. What a thrill to see any land. Soon it was announced on the loud speaker that we were in the Solomon Islands. On our right was Guadalcanal and to our left, San Cristobal. We stood at the railing to see this famous island so many brave men had died to secure. The branchless palms stood like sentinels against the sky, a grim reminder that only 18 months before, at a terrible human price, this small island had been reclaimed from the Japanese.

Now we were told where we were going! We were slated for New Guinea, the world's second largest island! There was a very nice commander among our passengers who had a book about the Pacific. We gathered around him as he read aloud to all of us about this place called New Guinea, a mountainous island inhabited by

Melanesians and by many animals similar to those in Australia since once, in the geological past, the two land forms had been connected. It was home to koala, small wallabies, lizards, snakes and many birds. Being part of the "Ring of Fire" there were frequent earthquakes. Southern New Guinea was Australian; Northern New Guinea was a Dutch territory.

We were headed for Milne Bay, on the southern tip of New Guinea, but we were diverted from Milne Bay by a bad storm. We were sent to Finschafen instead, on the southeast coast. We pulled into the harbor.

There was a flutter of semaphore. The "smart code" boys, who could read Morse Code in lights, told us the message had been "No Room. Go north!" We backed out of the harbor. Tension was high.

The loudspeaker blared, "WE WILL BE PASSING ENEMY TERRITORY TONIGHT!" (Wewak and Medang on the mid-east coast were still Japanese held.)

"YOU WILL CLOSE AND DARKEN YOUR PORTHOLES."

"THERE WILL BE NO LIGHTS - ZERO - THAT IS NO LIGHTS!"

"YOU WILL NOT SMOKE."

"THERE WILL BE NO NOISE!"

In the late twilight, we began our journey north along New Guinea's east coast, closer and closer to the Equator. We traveled as far out as we could so as not to become a perfect silhouette. We were blacked out, silent and fast. We were all tense.

That night we heard and saw our first ack-ack, not firing at us, but it was the first enemy fire we had heard. The rooms were stifling hot but we were blacked out and no one smoked or spoke above a whisper!

In the far distance we saw the outline of a rugged mountainous mass. We were told this backbone mountain chain was the Owen-Stanley Mountains.

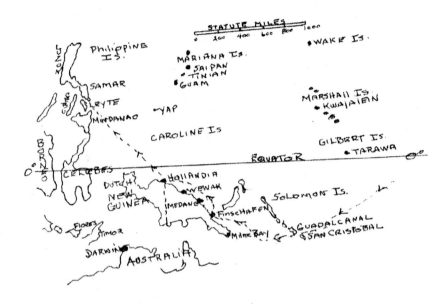

SOUTHWEST PACIFIC AREA — 1944

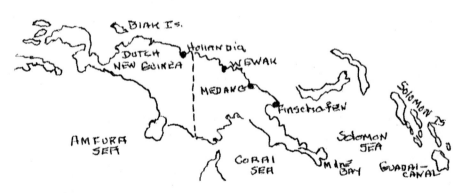

NEW GUINEA AND SURROUNDING ISLANDS — 1944

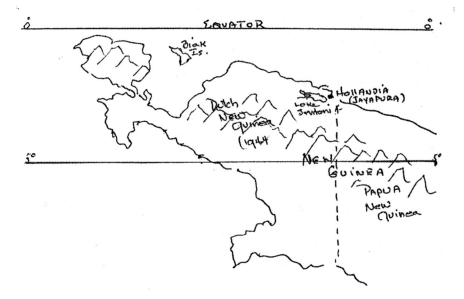

ENLARGEMENT OF DUTCH NEW GUINEA —
1944

CHAPTER THREE

Hollandia, New Guinea

First Impressions

Two days later we pulled into another harbor. Before us was Hollandia, in Dutch-owned New Guinea. Three months before, General Eichelberger's men had caught the Japs at breakfast here. We had held it since.

Shirl and I were topside early. Before us was a jungle island — steaming, hot, humid. We felt sorry for the guys who were to debark here.

The loud speaker blared, "All Nurses be ready to debark at 0730!" This was us! This was *our* destination — Hollandia, New Guinea (now Jayapura, Indonesia).

We all flew down to our quarters and packed up. We watched as our footlockers were heaved into a landing craft. One missed and went into the drink. It was mine. (It still smells moldy fifty years later.)

All of us were herded into an amazing machine — a "Duck." It took two of these amphibious craft to take us all. As we plowed to shore through Humboldt Bay, to a jetty (Pim Jetty) we saw small palm thatched huts on stilts standing in the water offshore. Smiling Melanesian people dressed in the most brilliant yellow and purple shirts were waving at us. We later learned these were GI shirts dyed with the commonly used drugs gentian violet and atabrine.

We waved to our companions on shipboard, then bravely faced this shore. Much to our amazement, our boats did not stop but rolled on wheels up the red-clay roadway, over the bank and sped along the narrow dusty road.

We were driving through what I now know was rain forest. To me then, it was a jungle — high trees and huge ferns like a carboniferous forest. A boar ran across the road in front of us. Cockatoos screamed from the treetops. They rose and settled as we passed.

How very strange it seemed to me coming from a cozy little New England town with green hills, warm valleys, white church spires, winding roads, friendly lakes, and fragrant fields of hay, to be here one degree below the equator on New Guinea in this dense jungle.

It was hot! It was humid. The "amphibious duck" was racing along through these green jungles passing smiling Melanesian people walking on the roads. There were jungle noises, birds, and insects. There was pungency in the smell of the moist, red soil mixed with the exhaust fumes from our vehicle. The road was narrow, but smooth. We learned that the Seabees had built this road above the wet jungle floor so well that supplies were easily transported to other facilities, whereas the Japanese had not been able to build well and had constant mud problems.

As we rounded a corner, there was a large, raw, newly bulldozed area just cleared of jungle, but still muddy and full of stumps. At the end of this clearing were two new barracks with cement floors, corrugated metal roofs with burlap suspended part way down from the eaves and up from the ground leaving a free space above and below.

"This is home, girls!" our smiling driver said as he pulled to a stop. We all piled out and stood dazed as he whirled his monster around and waved good-bye. It was Sunday morning, September 17, 1944. We had left Fort Devens August 21 and the States, August 27, 1944.

"Hi, where did you come from?" A very green-colored, attractive dark-haired girl came up to us, smiling.

"We just landed. We left Frisco in late August."

"How are things at home?" she asked, then happily explained her skin color. "Dark people get this color from atabrine. Blondes don't turn so dark." But she laughed and told us to check our hands. There it was. The yellow dye was starting to show.

The Germans had discovered atabrine, a real dye. They also discovered this dye could be used instead of quinine to control malaria. Most of the sources of quinine were in Southeast Asia and under Japanese control, so atabrine became our malarial prevention and control.

"Welcome to Hollandia and the 54th General! Take a bed inside. Be sure to use your mosquito nets and I'm afraid there is no latrine yet! You'll have to go by ambulance to the other end of the hospital for now!"

What a joke! Every time we had to go to the latrine, we had to take the ambulance. The guys driving us were so put out! "How do you answer your kids who ask, 'Hey Dad, what did you do to help win the war?' Answer: 'I drove nurses to the latrine in my ambulance!'"

Oh well, it didn't last too long.

That Sunday, when we arrived, we took a bed with a T-bar and put our suitcases and packs down. T-bars were attached to the head and the foot of each bed from which the mosquito netting was suspended. During the day the netting was rolled up and tied to the top bar. At night it was unrolled, attached to hooks on the bottom T-bar and our beds were encased in a bug-proof tent.

Shirl and I then went to a church service in a tent at the other end of this area. It was hot and sticky but it was a familiar service, and we enjoyed it. All through the service, I kept hearing a hot wire spit and crackle. No one else seemed to pay any attention, but I did and I was uncomfortable and anxious.

After the service I leaned forward to ask the soldier in front of me about the cause of the noise. He laughed, reached into a shrub by the tent and revealed a HUGE six-inch grasshopper. It was enormous. Both Shirl and I were impressed. We also learned that the GIs captured these creatures, tied one of the 'hopper's legs to their caps for a short time and then released the tie. The 'hoppers stayed on their caps like a feather decoration!

We were told everything was huge! The strange trees were very tall and they had small tufts of greenery on top. Their roots stood out like thin, curving, upright walls. I never learned what they were. Some of the seeds were six inches long. I tried to send home a flat, bean-like seed, but it never arrived.

There were orchids high in the trees and parasitic plants hanging in the treetops. Aside from the boar that ran in front of our amphibious duck that first day, the bats, the rats and the plentiful cockatoos, I saw no animal life, except for the python killed by the MPs as it was on its way across the nurses' area and headed through our barracks. It was 10-15 feet long. Knowing how plentiful the rats were, I'm sure he would have had good hunting. But I'm glad I did not have to confront him!

These very first days were strange. We lived in isolated barracks. It was so hot in the daytime, we couldn't do much but sit and either read or write or sleep. When we went to chow, we slogged across the newly-turned earth and picked up pounds of wet clay or gumbo on our shoes. We had to wear our long-sleeved shirts, long pants, wool socks and high shoes. By the end of mealtime, having braved the rains in our helmets and ponchos, we sat outside the barracks and scraped off five pounds of gumbo from each foot. This was "How soil is moved in New Guinea!"

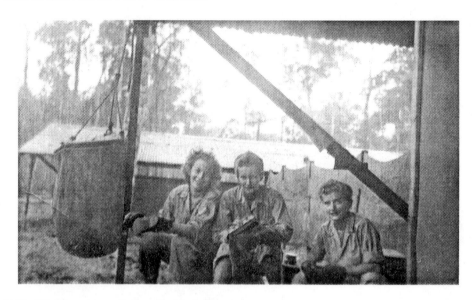

BC, Shirl, me and the lister bag.

When we wanted a drink, we went to the front of the barracks where, hanging in the sun, on a post was a lister bag. This was a rubberized, lined canvas bag (waterproof anyway) into which our drinking water was poured along with what tasted like chlorine. At any rate, this bag with its flavored, warm water was always available for drinking. It was really awful. Warm, rubberized, chlorinated water was not really exciting. But it was wet, so we drank it!

Life was fairly simple we found. We had to wash in our helmets. It was hard for more than undies. We went to the showers and latrines in the ambulance. By the second day, our quintumvirate decided to have an afternoon of fun and go back to the *Holbrook,* still in the harbor, and pay a visit. We had no orders to leave the base, no escort (all nurses were to have an armed escort, but we did not know this at the time) and no invitation. We were naive, stupid, and still civilians. We learned the hard way!

My letters home on this foolhardy expedition were incomplete, but the five of us got someone to take us to Pim Jetty, for a bribe of some beer, I think. Someone else carried us out deep into the harbor to that huge troop ship and we boarded through a cargo door.

Our former pals on the topside were stunned and not too pleased to see five 2nd lieutenants newly landed, now off the base with no orders, and no invitation to return! It was not long before five nurses and five innocent Naval officers were required to report at once to the captain's quarters!

September 21, 1944

Dear Folks,

… He was furious! He lectured us on Army discipline and the danger into which we put his ship, his officers, and ourselves to do such a stupid thing! He was forced to provide a boat to shore, to arrange an Army weapons carrier and a driver to take the five of us back to the hospital, but he also had to send us with the five armed Navy men we'd come to see, then return them to the shore and the ship. They were not happy with us. The Army was not happy with us. It was a terrible breach and mistake. We were so foolish and humiliated, and contrite! What we truly did not know, we learned very fast and very well and never forgot.

When the guys saw how we lived in our mud wallow they were appalled and wordless and were very grateful to get back to their clean ship. We had learned a terrible lesson.[3]

Never go anywhere or do anything without orders or permission! You're in the Army now!

Love, Sally B.

Staging—Hollandia

I remember —

In September of 1944, Hollandia, in Dutch New Guinea, was a huge staging[4] area for the 8th Army and the 7th Fleet. Having been taken from the Japanese in a successful surprise attack, there was not much destruction in evidence. When we sailed up the coast we saw the lovely green rugged spine of mountains, unbroken the whole length of the island. Humboldt Bay was a beautiful deeply-indented harbor with well-marked headlands on either side. Its arms were edged with unspoiled, sandy beaches shaded by overhanging palms.

Inland was the rain forest with huge tall trees, monstrous ferns and flashing birds. In the tall treetops were orchids. Intertwining the trees were net-like vines. Everything was damp and lush with a pungent smell.

---

[3] We never heard that we had been reported — so the captain never told. But we never forgot that lesson!
[4] Staging: A term for an area where personnel waiting to be assigned or deployed are gathered.

Through these jungles ran a beautiful gravel highway. Melanesian people, tall and straight, walked along the highway. We had first seen these people when we landed. They looked Negroid, but had sharper features and were not as dark. They were always clothed when we saw them. Their feet were usually bare, but some wore cast-off Army boots. Their legs were long and thin, so these boots were huge and made their legs look like toothpicks. They always smiled and seemed so good natured — but their smiles were different. Their teeth were often red from chewing betel nuts. That was a first for me. The children had lovely white teeth.

In the months we were there, I had no interaction with them. I knew some lived in Nipa huts built on stilts in the shallow water of the harbor. We had seen them when we landed. Others lived in similar Nipa huts in Lake Sentani. This was a large, beautiful lake about five miles inland that we were told had been an arm of the sea many years ago before being blocked by a lava flow. The lake was bordered by Army installations and some native huts.

Perhaps five or ten miles from the harbor, high above Lake Sentani, was a very important settlement of very important people.

There was a high hill located between the lake and the sea. On the top and high sides of this hill were 8th Army and 7th Fleet Headquarters, and most importantly, General MacArthur's headquarters. He lived there with his wife Jean, small son Arthur, and Arthur's nurse. We often saw General MacArthur and his family riding in his open car around the base nodding and waving. There

41

was a lot of anger at him among the men because he had his family with him, the only officer in the theater to have this honor. The men also resented the fact that they had only a beer issue and not the hard liquor all the officers seemed to have.

Just a note to add here — The GIs wanted hard liquor and couldn't get it, so many made their own called "jungle juice"! They hollowed out a coconut, added fruit and sugar and sealed it until the plug blew three times. Then it was ready!

I never tried it. It scared me. I heard a lot about the dangers of methyl alcohol and how it could kill a person.

Headquarters for both General Eichelberger, Commanding General of 8th Army (to which I was attached), and Admiral Halsey, Commander of the 7th Fleet, were both located on this hilltop. Quarters for staff officers of both the Army and Navy were located here also. They too were waiting.

Below, near Lake Sentani, was an airstrip from which early morning forays were made by our men flying the P-38s. They were our only bombers and had to make day flights because they could not fly at night. Our C-47 (DC-3s) supply planes were also based at this strip.

This lake area was the hub headquarters for many units — chemical engineers, Seabees, aviators, Australians, anti-aircraft and ancillary personnel of all kinds. Hollandia was also the site of two growing general hospitals: the 51st, located downhill from the base headquarters, and the 54th to which we were temporarily attached.

It was a bustling base. Everyone was waiting for our push north. On October 20, MacArthur invaded Leyte in the Philippines. The casualties began to come to Hollandia soon afterward.

During that first month, we became acclimated to equatorial heat, rain, mud, humidity and the wild life. We read, slept, and eventually found friends who were as ready for fun as we were. At this time, we were not allowed off our area without an armed escort. There were Japanese still in the mountains. Since we had no automobiles, there was no way we could get away from our hospital without an armed male officer companion.

September 27, 1944

Dear Folks,

Our barracks has developed into a cozy spot. Our footlockers are bureaus and desks, our beds are couches and refuge from the bugs. Off and on, we've had showers. When they are off, we use our helmets for baths. The only trouble is that washing shirts and pants in a helmet is a bit difficult. Life here is a real adventure.

We are not working yet, but heaven knows when we will — and we will. But getting used to equatorial climate is a challenge. Remember I told you my footlocker went in the drink? All my sheets, pillowcases, towels and clothes were soaked and stained, so one afternoon I washed everything in a pail.

One of my earliest victories here in the early weeks was my pail!

My friends and I went out with a group of Navy men who had a pailful of iced beer. When all the beer was gone, I asked for the pail. My date was so happy he was glad to give it to me. SO, I became the owner of #1 wash basin!! So many gals want to use the pail to wash in that I have to hang a sign-up list daily for 30 minute intervals.[5]

Showers are not too private either. They are open at the top so any buzz-boy can swoop low over us while we are getting clean and bother us a bit. One of our nurses has a fiancé who does this. We all know it is Junior. Just fun.

The food is good, monotonous but well prepared, considering what they have to work with. I'm not too hungry. It's too hot. I sit around all day—write letters and play bridge.

Twice now I've been out with a man in Naval Intelligence. His name is Hank and he's from Connecticut. He is so pleasant and such a gentleman. Tomorrow he's taking Shirl and me on a sightseeing tour of the island. We are excited, for Hollandia is a beautiful spot, beautiful mountains, harbors and jungle scenery. I'll write you.

Our nurses are fine. We get along well! We laugh a lot. It helps to spend the hours. Shirl and I sent home a lot of heavy clothes. No need for them here!

Love, Me

---

[5] I carried that pail with me until the day I left to come home.

September 28, 1944

Dear Mom and Dad,

... Sightseeing with Hank was a real experience. First time I went out with him, we went for a picnic at See-wee-gee Beach next to the big bay. It was beautiful there with a wide unspoiled sandy beach with palms drooping over us. Hank and I went wading. It was a picture of tropical magic with palms, sand and the push and pull of the gentle waves. It's so hard to think of ships of war out there somewhere and I know they are. Hank is a very nice person and very much a gentleman.

The second time I saw him, he took Shirley, one of his friends, and me sightseeing. Before taking us to his headquarters for supper, he took us to several landing strips strewn with wrecked ZEROS — small Japanese fighter planes.

From 7th Fleet Headquarters the view of the mountains, Lake Sentani and lovely clouds and shadows is magnificent. It was a delicious meal and Shirl and I felt happy to have met these two men who were so helpful and who introduced us to this faraway area!

We have a bit of humor here too. Over our latrine is a huge gum tree. We now have a six-holer under a tent protected by a roll of burlap on the sides. There is little privacy, but it beats being taken to the latrine in the ambulance!!

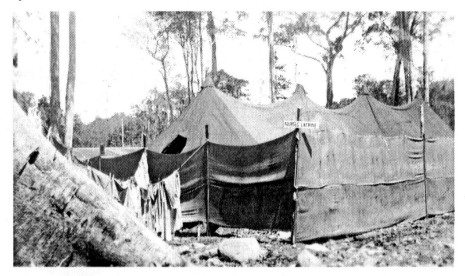

Our first latrine where we were serenaded by the musical bird.

In that gum tree sits a lovely bird that sings the first two measures of "Bell Bottom Trousers." At first, since there were so many guys all walking around our area that, as I said, was pretty crude, we were embarrassed, thinking they were able to see us. Then we found out what we were hearing was a bird! He's lovely, like a parrot. Our men would never do that to us!!

No mail yet, but since it took us three weeks to get here, I'm sure mail will come sometime! We long to hear from everyone at home! ...

Love, Sally B.

October 9, 1944

Dear Grampus,

... Here we are in the middle of a new hospital getting built. It has grown rapidly since we came. The trees are palms and gums and there are huge ferns. In the tops of the trees are the parasites called "birds nests." The tree trunks seem to be enlaced with netting. Wish I had a book to tell me what I'm seeing. (strangler figs?)

I still have trouble believing I'm here. The only thing that jerks me back to my senses is that, while we drive along, the men, women and children are all decked out in the queerest clothes combinations from GI trousers to some bright rag, which had been someone's shirt. The women carry large bundles on their heads while the men walk behind, looking around, smiling, waving and even hitchhiking along the road. They look like our Negroes, only smaller and I'm afraid, quite dirty.

As yet we have not worked, but we are waiting! Some nurses have been over here many months, so our few weeks are nothing.

I think of you often and look forward to some more of our wonderful talks. I miss them.

Much love, Sally B.

October 12, 1944

Dear Mom and Dad,

At last we got mail. I got 37 letters! I sat down to sort them by date and then had a field day. It was wonderful. Everyone perked up and was happy.

How wonderful to get news of the new trees and the garden and all the canning you two are doing in your new home. It was wonderful to get the pictures of the house and garden and you two. I'm trying to get some pictures here and I'll send what I can.

I've been very social. It helps to break the routine. Sometimes it's fun. Many times it is a strain. It is so hard on everyone to be waiting. Everyone needs and wants someone to care for, to hold on to. But we do not want to be that one. Lots of anxiety in everyone who is waiting.

Love, Me

October 18, 1944

Dear Mom and Dad,

… Today I had a wonderful time! Eight of us went swimming, just like Greensboro, Vermont, full-blown play, jumping, pushing, and diving — all followed by turkey sandwiches. Such a lovely day. I'm as red as a beet and tons will peel off, but we all had such a good time.

Love, Sally B.

Move to Tent City

October 19, 1944

Dear Mom and Dad,

… We've moved again to a staging area across the road from the hospital. We are now in a tent village with four of us in each tent. BC, Shirl, Knowlsey and I are in one. Mickey's right next door. The floors are dirt and we sleep on canvas cots. But we've fixed up our new home. Our cots are along the sides, our footlockers are our bureaus and we hang our clothes around the edges of the tent. It's really camping out. One light bulb hangs from the center pole. We have latrines and showers. The latrine is a 16-holer, each with a wooden cover and heart shaped hole! It is screened and has a door with a half moon and a sign, which says "Private."

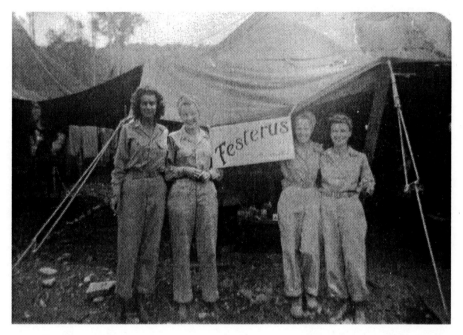

Shirl, BC, Knowlsey and me in front of our tent "Festerus" in Tent City.

The showers are special with separate compartments for showers, huge sinks to wash in and benches to put things on. So nice to keep clean. I tend to soak through three changes every day, so my laundry is big enough! I use my pail to do my laundry in. It is a wonderful thing to have.

We have to wear high shoes, wool socks, our tan pants and shirts all the time. At night our sleeves must be rolled down, our collars buttoned high. It is for mosquito control. Can't remember when I wore a dress.

We now are under a new command, a new organization. Our whole tent village is casuals. We have a new commander and a swell chief nurse. So our temporary duty with the 54th General is over. Soon we will be assigned.

We've named our tent in the new tent city "Festerus" (a Navy term for a "thingamabob"). Each of our group has named her tent. Our neighbors have "Duffy's Tavern," next is "Copley Plaza." Our roadway is Holbrook Blvd. We've staked our claim on our small area in Hollandia!

Love, Sally B.

I remember —

Unbeknownst to my cohorts and me at the time, on October 20 our troops had landed in Leyte in the Philippines. We were kept in the dark about all troop movements. All we knew was that Hollandia was full of medical personnel and special Navy and Army people who, like us, were waiting.

October 24, 1944

Dear Folks,

… As for my adventures in New Guinea, they have broadened considerably this past week. BC, Shirl and I have met some "Buzz Boys" flyers, Bud, Bob and Tater. They took us flying!! Bud was the pilot of a C-47. We flew for an hour and a half over this beautiful area. It was like a dream to fly over the green mountains. There were clouds below and all around us, catching the reflection of the setting sun. I had always dreamed about flying through a cloud and we were doing it. Bud let each of us fly the plane for a bit. Of course, it was a hoax. He never let go for long.

As we flew over the trees, flocks of cockatoos rose up like clouds of popcorn. We saw the bay,[6] the lake, the hospital. What an adventure.

I don't know how Bud got permission to take us up. We burned a lot of gas. But I'll never forget. These young men were the ones who introduced us to Australians in the next camp. One afternoon we were eating sandwiches or having a beer at Bud's, Bob's and Tater's camp when several men in shorts and cocked brimmed hats dropped in. It was the first time I'd heard an Aussie speak. It was a challenge. I remember asking many questions about Australia, the kangaroos and koalas. They told us a lot about a country about which I knew so little. They told us about the terrible Japanese bombing of Darwin.

---

[6] I took a picture of Humboldt Bay, but didn't realize it had so many ships in it until it was developed. I hid it in my suitcase 'till I got home.

We learned where so many of our supplies came from. They told us about Sydney and its beautiful harbor.

(It would be many years before I saw Sydney, and it was as beautiful as these men told us it was.)

On another evening, a group of us were asked to a party given by 8th Army Ordinance. Most of the men were majors, lieutenant colonels, and colonels. They were very pleasant. I met two geologists from whom I got answers to many of my questions about this area.

The next day, the same group of us went on General Eichelberger's yacht for a trip around the bay. What a lovely spot. I had a great talk with a young man who had traveled extensively in Alaska as well as in large areas in this theater. There is much of the world to see! I'd love to go to see more of our world someday.

When we landed, we had supper and spent a lovely evening by the lake playing bridge and drinking pineapple juice. My date was Dick T. in chemical warfare. He was so pleasant and kind. It was a lovely day. The only thing that really jarred me was that these officers all seem to have individual iceboxes in their quarters when many of the hospital wards have to use boxes filled with ice which originally were used to refrigerate blood. I found this most upsetting and not right! Maybe I don't understand all the thinking behind this observation, but this is what I saw and did not like.

Love, Me

October 28, 1944

Dear Mom and Dad,

… Shirl and I have latrine detail every morning now, cleaning and scrubbing our facilities. We all have jobs to police the area, but Shirl and I got this first. It's not the most pleasant, but it has to be done like we used to clean bedpans in nursing school. It's a good feeling to leave the area all spruced up and shining.

Just a note more about our tent. It's really homey now. We use my pail upside down as a seat under the light to write letters. We found half a log that I put next to the pole under the light bulb, with a bottle with a candle in it and our books standing near the candle. There we are! We have a little home!

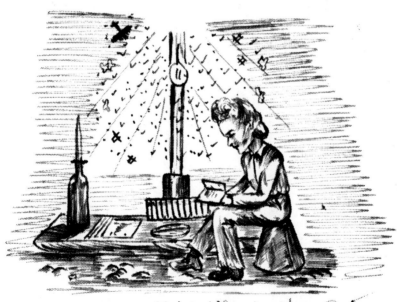

Night life in New Guinea

We made up a song to the tune of "Mother"

G - is for the gnats there are to plague us

U- is for the uselessness we feel

I - is for the Iodine extension (code word for our phone line here)

N- is for the nets that do us shield

E - is for the everlasting mud holes

A - is for the atabrine we take (and I am yellow)

Put them all together they spell Guinea

The place we hope we'll all forsake!

One night it had been pouring rain. We'd been out and came into the tent and turned on the light bulb. Many rats ran in every direction across our dirt floor. That was very disagreeable. And we remembered the hunting expedition of the killed python. Good hunting for him! Mickey was bitten by a rat one night. Great excitement by all the group of medical people and all of us!

Love, Sally B.

November 2, 1944

Dear Mom and Dad,

… Time is flying by. I can't believe it was over a week ago I wrote, but this resort life is something, especially for us who are not yet working. Rumor has it we will be soon. We all hope it means we will be going to the Philippines soon!

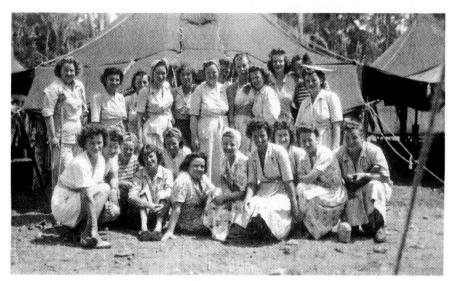

The casual gang — back row, left to right: Dottie, Helen, Mary, Ruthie, Bernice, Edna, Barky, Roz, Myrt, Shirl, Rainey, and Ballou. Front row, left to right: Irene, Irish, Knowlsey, Mary, Dottie, Mickey, BC, Tommy, Juney, Milly, and Gahagan. Some are missing.

Remember I wrote that some pilots had taken us flying? Last week, BC, Shirl and I went surf boarding on the lake with them. One of the guys had obtained a motorboat from the Navy and had made a surfboard. Everyone tried, as did I. It is a bit like skiing and it took me a while to catch on, but I finally did it. I felt so proud!

Following our surfboard fun on the lake, there was a base order NEVER to swim in the lake again. It seems that the natives who live in Nipa huts that stand on pilings in the water at the edge of the lake have YAWS, a spirochete infection. The water was unclean because of many things, but it had been such fun. Of course, we will *never* go again.

Three days ago we had an exciting experience. Some of us were hanging out clothes when a strangely silent oriental-looking man came near, sat and stared, didn't speak or move. Eerie! One of the gals went for an MP. This was a starving Japanese soldier who had been cut off from supplies for weeks. We knew there were Japanese in the hills. This was the reason we had to go out with *armed* officers at night. His tour was over!

… Last night I went up to 7th Fleet Headquarters to a party with a Navy flyer. My date neither smoked nor drank which was nice. He is the copilot on Admiral Kincaid's B-24. He loves that plane and enjoyed talking about it to me. Then he offered to take me through it. Who am I to refuse?!

It is like a Pullman car with tables, chairs, two heads, clothes closets, all sorts of gadgets and earphones by each chair.

I said, "This plane has everything but the kitchen sink!" Then I saw it — a chrome and aluminum sink and shelves and an electric icebox.

Cal took me into the cockpit to show me everything. I sat in the pilot's seat, heard "Beethoven's 6th" over the earphones from Tokyo, saw the board under fluorescent lighting for night work. It was awesome! I was amazed and humbled when I realized brother John flies this same plane whose dash lights look like San Francisco at night! How pleasant this evening was!

Love, Me

November 6th, 1944

Dear Folks,

... We had a terrible windstorm today. Our tent almost blew down. We held on to our ropes like fury, but our tent poles had to be reset and our tent realigned.

I'm enclosing a picture of me trying to read on my pail with P-38 and F6F-like bugs whirling by, skidding on my pages and leaving tracks as they go. Finally gave up and crawled into my mosquito netting and went to sleep.

It's wonderful to get news of home. You have no idea how precious each letter is!

Love, Sally B.

November 13, 1944

Dear Mom and Dad,

... It's been a busy week for me, sewing, reading, sketching, and an amazing event has occurred. I met an anti-aircraft captain who knows another Sally Hitchcock and her brother Peter who live in Columbus, Ohio.

I had heard of the other Sally Hitchcock when I was a junior at Smith College. It seems that she had graduated some years ahead of me from Smith with a major in anthropology or archeology.

There was a major mix up somewhere when I received a letter from a museum in Boston thanking me for my interesting exhibit on Indian corn! I knew this was a BIG mistake! The name was the same, but the topic was all wrong. I remember writing to the museum to tell them I was not the person in question. That was when I discovered this other woman with the same name as mine who had graduated a few years ahead of me.

Do you know of this Ohio family, Dad? Are we related? I know many Connecticut families went west to the Western Reserve in Ohio.

He saw my name and was shocked, so he looked me up. He's very nice and we have a fine time talking. His name is Val.

Thank you Dad, for forwarding copies of John's letters. What a relief to know he is OK. It's been months since I heard from him. And I'm so glad he's home for now. How relieved you must be!

I'm enclosing my diary in pictures. Please save them because I have so few camera shots.

Love, Me

A Diary in Pictures
Sent home for safekeeping in mid-November 1944

Memoirs of New Guinea

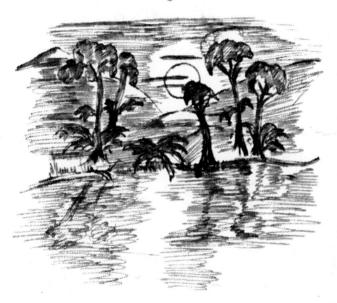

First Impressions

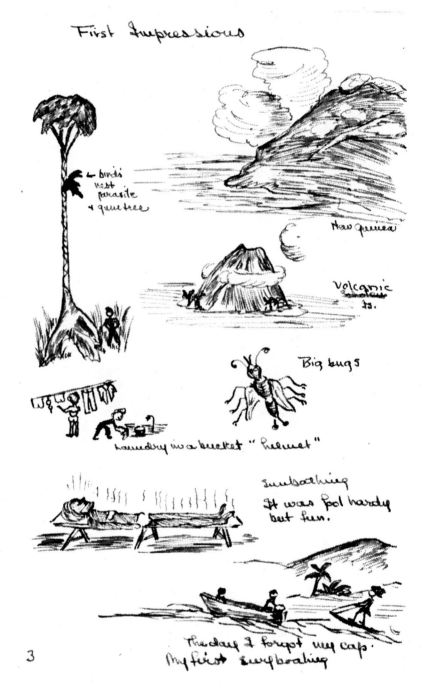

← bird's nest parasite + gum tree

New Guinea

Volcanic I.

Big bugs

Laundry in a bucket "helmet"

Sunbathing
It was fool hardy but fun.

The day I forgot my cap.
My first surfboating

3

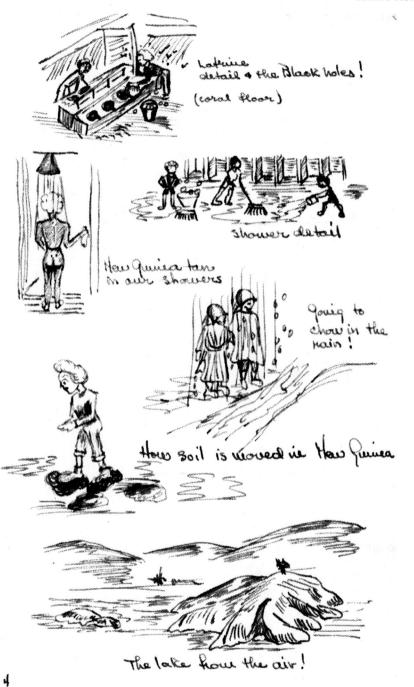

Latrine detail & the Black holes! (coral floor)

shower detail

New Guinea tans in our showers

Going to chow in the rain!

How soil is moved in New Guinea

The lake from the air!

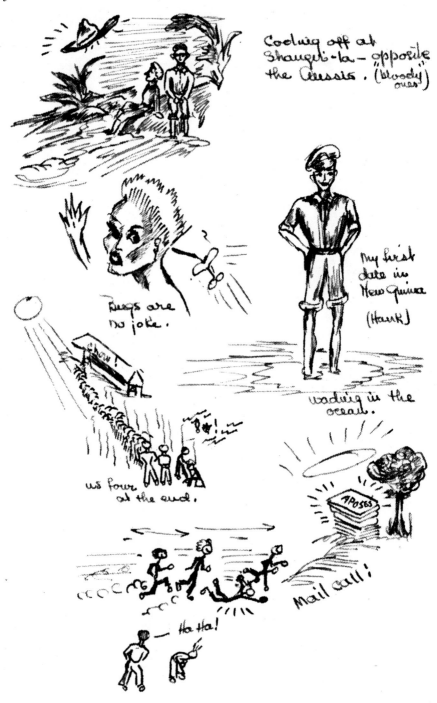

Cooling off at Shangri-la — opposite the Aussies. ("bloody" ones)

Jeeps are no joke.

My first date in New Guinea (Hank)

wading in the ocean.

us four at the end.

APO 565

Mail call!

Ha Ha!

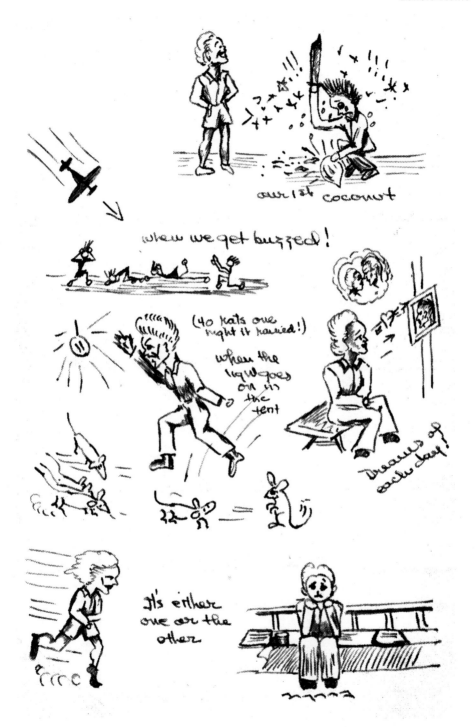

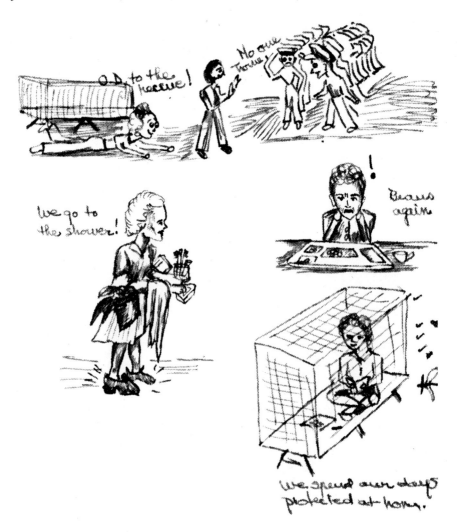

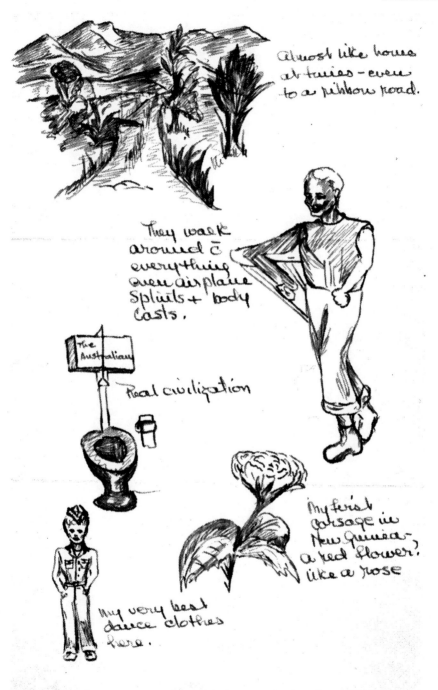

Almost like home at times - even to a ribbon road.

They walk around c̄ everything even airplane splints + body casts.

The Australian

Real civilization

My first corsage in New Guinea - a red flower? like a rose

My very best dance clothes here.

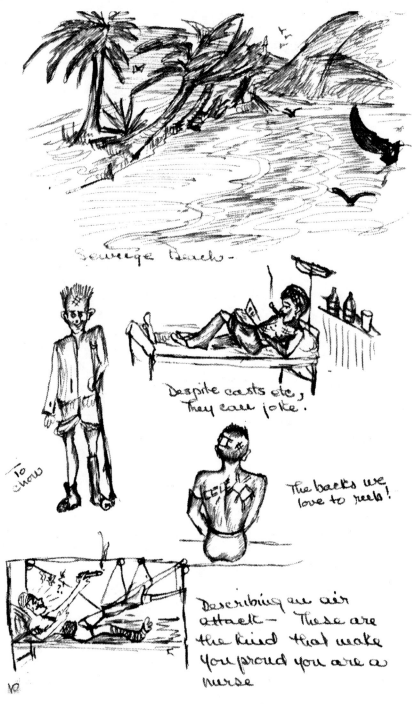

Sewage Beach -

To chow

Despite casts etc, They call joke.

The backs we love to reeb!

Describing an air attack - These are the kind that make you proud you are a nurse

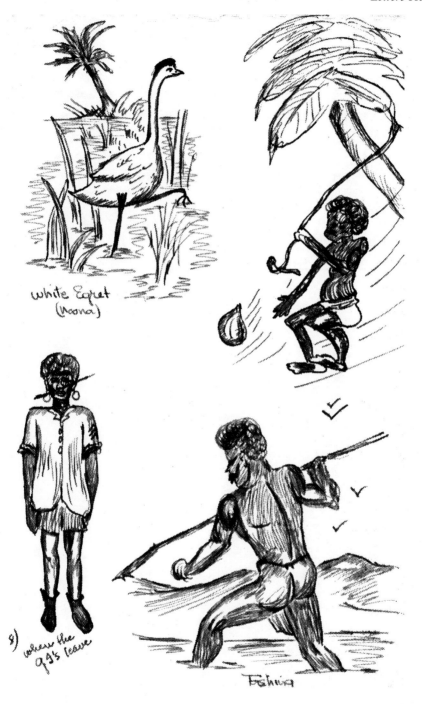

white Egret
(noona)

9)
when the
gg's leave

Fishing

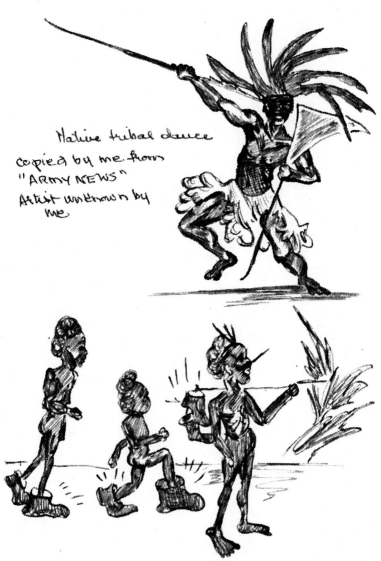

Native tribal dance copied by me from "ARMY NEWS" Artist unknown by me.

9) The natives wake a haul where the GI's pull out — (like pipe cleaners in to league boots!

(I drew this one.)

Detached Service
54th General Hospital

November 18, 1944

Dear Mom and Dad,

… Victory at last. We went to work!!

Yesterday for the first time some of us were put on temporary service at the 54th General where we were ensconced when we first came, before we were put over in our tent city. I was put on Officers' Surgery. Most of these men are casualties from Leyte.

It has been ages since I worked and I was nervous. The nurses in charge didn't give me an assignment so I went around to see what there was to do. One man asked me to change his dressing. I did and I relaxed. Then I took all the temps, passed out water, rubbed backs, straightened sheets, the old "P.M. Care" routine.[7]

I was busy. The men were pleased, and so my first work day in New Guinea passed!

Play time is short now. Full workdays fill my time and I'm tired. Val, the captain, who knows the other Sally Hitchcock, is nice. We sit around with his friends and talk and laugh. It's comfortable. He's thoughtful. He brought my three roommates and me pillows because we had none. We'd been using clothes stuffed in the pillowcases. He brought us a water can so we'd have drinking water in our tent. Even though he's been here many months, he is still generous and kind and unspoiled.

---

[7] P.M. Care was a procedure taught early in nurses' training — a late afternoon routine to make the patients more comfortable.

It's pouring again and the wind is fierce. I hate to slog up to work all muddy, but c'est la guerre!!

Not much other news except Anne is still in Hawaii and on nights. Thanks for buying that bond for me, Dad …

Love, Sally B.

I recall —

One of my memories not in a letter was of an event on that Officers' Ward where I was doing detached service. I've never forgotten it. I was handing out basins for back and hand washes, and back rubs. Since this was my only assignment, I went down the left 15 beds to the end, washing, rubbing backs and straightening sheets.

Across from the last patient on the left was a black officer. I crossed to him to do his care when his left hand neighbor (an officer) said, "Don't touch me after you've done him!" Such terrible racial prejudice! I was shocked. The ward was suddenly silent. I turned to him and said, "I won't!" I did special care to the black officer and skipped the offending person. I was angry. I could have made a speech, but didn't. I went right up the right-hand row of beds and finished. How terribly unfair and unkind and SMALL!

Next afternoon I had the same assignment. There were no comments from anyone and I did everyone with no comments.

At this time I was unaware that there was so much segregation and discrimination in the Army, I only knew about the Navy.

Detached Service
51st General Hospital

November 24, 1944

Dear Mom and Dad,

Today is your Thanksgiving. What a wonderful day you all must have had with John home and safe. I can just picture all the fruit in the little wooden wagon on the dining room table, turkey, gravy, mashed potatoes, with celery and carrots and squash and onions and pumpkin and mince pies.

It was a different day for me. Shirl, BC, Knowlsey and I were transferred from "Festerus" and the 54th to the 51st General, past our airstrip. We're on detached service again. I hated to leave, but here we are.

Just before I left my Officers' Ward, I watched the colonel give out purple hearts. The guys joked and laughed but they were proud deep inside just the same. They were fine officers and gentlemen. I was deeply touched.

The Army gave us 12 hours to pack up over night. We were to be ready at 0900 Thanksgiving morning. We were ready when our friend Val came with a jeep and a trailer and took us lock, stock and barrel to this hillside hospital.

It's like a palace here compared to our tent village. We have real beds with mattresses and pillows. There are washing machines, real showers, isolated nurses' quarters with cement floors. And we have flush johns! There's a big tank up high with a pull chain. How very civilized!!

My work here is on a surgical floor of enlisted men, all banged up in Leyte. Most are Army but we have Navy men too. This is a plastic surgical floor, so there are many dressings and treatments to do.

Behind us on the mountaintop are MacArthur's Headquarters, 8th Army and those of the 7th Fleet. Below us are the airstrip and the lovely Lake Sentani. If we had to be anywhere, this is a pretty special place to be.

We are very busy! When I first came here, I would help the doctors with these daily dressings and irrigations. Now special teams of doctors and nurses from this 51st General go north in 48-hour shifts to help on the front in field hospitals. The teams rotate, but this leaves *big* holes where doctors and nurses have been removed. We have to do what they had been doing. Every day I thank God for all the training I received, my operating room months, my surgery and all the theory I have had, because I was asked to do things I've never done and there is no one else to do them.

We all work very hard. It is so hot that I'm usually wringing wet after an hour, but we're all getting used to it!

Guess I'm a wee bit homesick tonight, but it will pass. Hope you enjoyed the sketches. 'Twas fun and a way to share my world with all of you at home. It's 10:00 p.m. and I'm tired, I've worked eight hours and I've done a big wash. What a joy a washing machine is!!

Love, Me

November 30, 1944

Dear Folks,

… We are working so terribly hard. I'm glad I can, but I don't have time to sit to write long letters. Thanks so much for pictures of the gang at home.

Two days ago I got the most wonderful present. Val made me a combination bureau and desk. It's a desk on one end and it has a space for my bureau with lots of shelves, so I do not have to live out of my suitcase. What a lovely thing to do. He is so thoughtful. (*I had that special furniture with me until the day I left the Philippines*)

A patient gave me a necklace made of shells and a matching bracelet. He's a good sport. Now I have four bracelets, a letter opener made of a 31-caliber Jap shell, a clip of 25mm Jap shells and six packages of Japanese cigarettes. Some day I'll deliver all these in person …

Love, Me

December 4, 1944

Dear Mom and Dad,

…Working, working and in two weeks I'm to go on nights, then our detached service will end and all of us casuals will become staff for the 126th General Hospital! Going north very soon. It's so good to know we will belong to something and that all of our wonderful group will be together again!

I met a lad here, Anthony Barkowski from Mellon Street in Bristol, Connecticut (*the town where I was born and brought up*). He's so nice. I also met a very young lad from Brattleboro, Vermont (*where my parents retired*). He is Hender Dye, so young and now healing from wounds he got at Leyte. We've had some fun talks about Vermont. You might call his Mom and tell her he's well and what a fine young (he's 18) man he is. Tomorrow he goes back to his outfit.

Saturday night I went to a wonderful party. We had roast beef, veal, cucumber and tomato salad and fresh lettuce and ice cream. It was a Real Event. My date was the nice Major Dick T. (chemical warfare) who made the aluminum wrist watch band for me. The mess hall was the dance hall and was all decorated by the natives with Kunai Grass (*a tall grass with long fluffy seeds on the top*). Oriental lanterns were everywhere. We had a 14-piece orchestra!!

I met several officers from Australia, the Netherlands, and Java. One Javanese general was smaller than I!

Dick filched a red hibiscus blossom for me and I wore it on my shirt. Shirl and I had our pictures taken with the "brass" in our very best dance clothes, high-necked, long-sleeved shirts, long pants, wool socks, high shoes!! The picture with all those officials, generals, governors, was printed in the Army News. And I was reprimanded for being out of uniform! It was the flower! Oh, well …

Love, Me

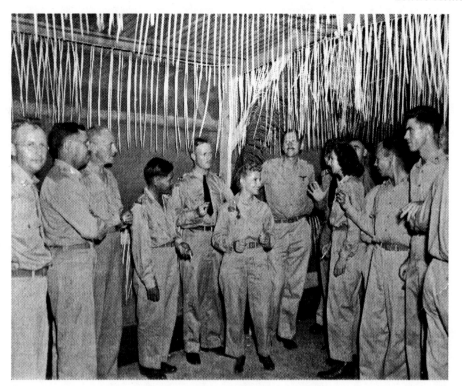

Left to Right: Unknown, Col. Thayer, Lt. Gen. Van Oyen, Col. Abdulkader, Lt. Westerman, Lt. Sally Hitchcock, Capt. Norquette, Lt. Gov. Gen. Dr. Van Nook, Lt. Shirley Munson, Maj. Tanner and Captain Welch.

I remember —

This is a funny story. For one split second, this arrangement of people made a good picture. It did not last. We all moved on, I with my date Dick T. and Shirl with her date. A trick of fate made a great "photo op!"

December 9, 1944

Dear Mom and Dad,

How happy I was to get your letters of the 19th of November and to know you both, John and Grampus will share Thanksgiving. It's good to stop worrying about John for a while now he's home.

An amazing event occurred today! Several of us were hanging out our wash on the line. You remember we have washing machines. It's nice. The chow line is close to our clothesline. We noticed several dark-haired men in uniforms quite unlike any we'd seen before standing at the end of the chow line.

One of our group went for the MPs again. Several appeared. These soldiers were terribly hungry Japanese left stranded as our Army units cut them off. They had turned themselves in. This is the second time we've turned in hungry Nip soldiers.

No packages yet, but never hesitate to send food, Triscuits, condensed milk, cookies, candies, canned meats, soup, coffee, cocoa, nuts and popcorn. Use this letter as a request if you have to. We can pop corn in our mess kits. It's so good.

I'm so glad to be working. I have 40 patients. There are two of us, plus the ward men. Yesterday we had to share nurses because of the teams who are gone, so we are real short. There is so much to do. I never thought I'd be able to probe and dig and scrub open wounds. You have to do it. In one draining wound, I probed and pulled out a piece of shrapnel. Some rewards anyway. You keep a stiff upper lip and so do the men, but it's emotionally draining to see such wounds.

All we can do is help heal them. These guys are brave! I'm so fond of them. They are so young! The other day I was working on a very young sailor who had been all shot up. He was depressed saying he'd never get up again. I laughed and said, "Of course you will." I cut up a shoe for his good foot and found him some crutches. He looked aghast and said he couldn't.

I was back after supper for back rubs. He was up, all smiles, "Hey, Lieutenant, I did it!" He was beaming. Today he came wobbling after me, "Hey, Sally, if you'll put the alcohol bottle under my arm, I'll carry it for you!" He was 19 yesterday. They are all so young!

Another patient had his left hand amputated. He's gutsy. He always smiles and jokes and does everything for himself. Yesterday I was doing dressings on his legs and we got to talking. He had been accepted into Harvard Medical School, then got drafted. 'Well," he said, "I was lucky to get off with no bodily injuries!" I encouraged him to realize how much he could do with one hand and a prosthesis on the other. At least he'll go home! What a spirit!

Much activity is going on around and near us. Every morning we hear the P-38s take off from the strip below us. We have gotten so we count them as they take off, then count them as they come back. We can hear trouble and we know we'll have patients. Plastic surgery is always a challenge, it's so long term.

Two special patients I will never forget. One is a very young sailor who has a huge area missing behind his knee. The two large tendons are there, but not much else. The void is full of sulfa powder.

I am upset by this wound, but so as not to react too much, I eat no breakfast.

About 30 minutes before I plan to do his care, I medicate him for pain then go back to do irrigations and packs done previously by the doctor. This lad looks at me, I'm sure he wonders how I take his infirmity and whether I know what I am doing. He is to be boarded home for a lot of grafting, but he is a really gutsy guy.

Then there is Tom B. with multiple gunshot wounds and many pieces of shrapnel still in his legs. He has a wound that goes diagonally all the way through his thigh. We have to probe it from both sides to keep it open to heal from the inside out. When there is no longer a doctor to do this, I have to do it.

The shrapnel sticking out of his leg caught on the sheets so I was told to remove the pieces, to do the best I could. There were no doctors available at this time. I washed the areas, made a nick with a scalpel, and removed the slivers. Washing carefully with azochloromide, I fired some butterflies[8] and closed the wounds. They are healing well. I am pleased.

Love, Sally B.

---

[8] Handmade adhesive closures had to be sterilized (fired) over an open flame.

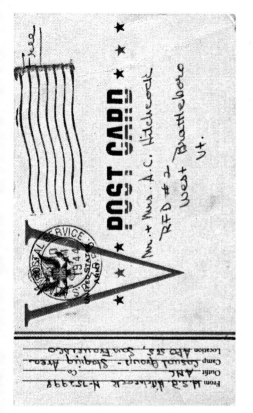

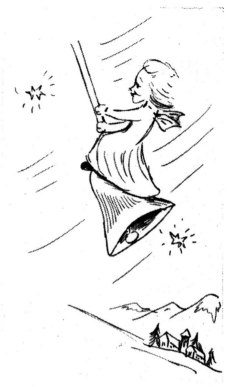

My Christmas card home on a V-Mail penny postal.

December 19, 1944

Dear Mom and Dad,

... Surprise! I find I'm scheduled for nights again. It's my second assignment on nights: I'm so mad. I was supposed to go to a big party at Naval Headquarters. Henry Fonda was to be there! I was to go with the Navy officer who had written all the songs for the Princeton Triangle shows. He's nice and fun and I wanted to go. Guess my wings were clipped.

Oh, well, nights will be a challenge. I just wish I could sleep days, but it's so hot. I'm thinking of Christmas at home, the balsam smells, the lovely red candles, the perfect little tree and my last trip home on that long, crowded train from New Haven. It was so cold and I was so hungry and tired.

Remember the long taxi ride I had around Brattleboro? It was crowded with many of us trying to make Christmas. Since I lived so far out in the country, everyone else sharing the taxi was let out first. Remember you told me the charming elderly taxi passenger who offered me a ride in his taxi was Ambassador Bunker? How warm and friendly he was! But my home was finally there with the candles in the windows. How cold it was! You, Mom, opened the door and there were the greens in the hall with red bows. We had the traditional pork, peas and red applesauce. The fire was snapping in the fireplace.

Here I sit battling bugs — P-38s, B-17s B-29s with huge stingers, "wings like a bat, almost as big as a cow and much meaner" is what my ward men say!!

A Navy man I knew on the *Holbrook*, Dick M., came for a visit tonight. He stayed about two hours. He's a very decent and kind person. Merry Xmas folks!

Much love, Me.

December 22, 1944

Dear Mom and Dad,

… Nights are not too bad. I have four wards and eight ward men, two to a ward. Each ward holds 40 patients but our census is very low. I have the 7 p.m. to 7 a.m. shift. It is long and between 2 and 5 a.m., it is hard to stay awake.

Nighttime is hard for these men who are patients. They can't sleep. One-by-one they come up and talk to me if I'm not busy. They worry about their homes, the wives they have and don't know, kids they have never seen, parents who are elderly, pals they've lost. They verbalize about the horrors of the war they have been in and how scared they were and how little they want to go back. A young man (18 years), Hender Dye, of Brattleboro, came up and we got acquainted before he shipped out. A nice young man, so very young, injured in Leyte.

Slowly the wards are emptied. We have either sent them back to duty all well or shipped them stateside for long-term care. These guys are wonderful. They have helped me days, helped each other and now most are gone. So, my census is very low. Only 40 convalescent patients! Easy! Duck Soup!

Love, Sally B.

December 27, 1944

Dear Mom and Dad,

... This is quite a tale, being on duty Christmas Eve. In the afternoon, BC and I went to Val's and with his friends we popped corn and had fun talking. Those guys are so nice. Then we came home and BC and I toasted your Triscuits and nuts, had a Nestle chocolate drink. That was our Christmas Eve feast. Thanks to all your goodies, we had a real party. I made a red paper carnation and put it in my buttonhole. "Out of Uniform!" I can hear it now, but it was Christmas Eve.

This night I will NEVER forget. Among the officers of the 51st, there was a party going on. All the medical, nursing and day staff, many of whom had served for weeks rotating to the front in 48 hour shifts, were celebrating. They were exhausted but back in Hollandia. It was a fun time to relax and enjoy. The patient load was small and not severely sick, so the party began early. I reported for my duty at 7 p.m. – December 24. I went on, checked my four wards. All was quiet.

But at 7:30 p.m. came the fatal phone call:

"ALL BEDS WILL BE FILLED. HOSPITAL SHIP UNLOADING AND AMBULANCES ENROUTE!"

I had 80 empty beds! You can not believe how we hustled getting all units ready to receive litter-borne men. All the ward men and the ambulatory patients were given jobs to see that each unit was supplied with a chart, pitchers (empty until we were sure the patient could drink), clean equipment, and towels. We were in a flurry of activity.

The men began to arrive. Some were so very sick! Many still had TAT (Tetanus Anti-Toxin) written on their foreheads in black ink. They were still dirty, some in their uniforms, having been given first aid and sent along. Dressings were dirty. IVs needed renewing. The sickest were placed on the ward I'd been serving on days.

I rushed to list the sickest ones so the doctor could see them first, then slowly all 80 beds were filled on my four wards. With everyone's help the men were put into beds, cleaned up the best we could, given food and water if no wounds were internal and I waited for the doctor to come.

But when he finally came, he had been celebrating too long and too hard. I called my supervisor. Everyone was swamped. She could send me no more help.

"Do the best you can," she said. So, I made rounds with the doctor. He was not at his best and a problem for me and for the men who were hurt, but at least I did get a blanket order for dressing changes and IVs and narcotics. Thank Yale for its training. I was able to function.

I was able to change dressings and clean up these very sick men. We medicated all that needed pain meds to help them rest. Every ward man was wonderful. So were all the ambulatory men. We all helped each other and somehow we quieted and cleaned the sickest ones, then moved to the other three wards where there was need but which was not so acute.

What a night! Somehow I managed to get through. The men were clean and resting. I was able to chart on everyone and accounted for all my narcotics but one half grain of codeine. A miracle.

Early Christmas morning, I took the big box of maple sugar hearts you had sent to me and put one heart on each bedside stand in the sick ward. It was a fun way to say '"Merry Christmas!"

Early, before morning report, the ward officer doctor of the night before arrived to see his patients! He had to rewrite some of the orders he'd written the night before. He was so contrite. Nothing awful had happened to his patients, but he and they and I were very glad for a new beginning. The chief nurse congratulated me on a job well done!

I had to go back on duty Christmas night. It was a breeze compared to the night before. I could hardly believe we all had survived that night. (*I know now that never in all the years that followed was there ever a bigger challenge! Anything that was asked after Christmas Eve was nothing in comparison!!*)

I was glad to start to bed on the morning of the 26th of December, but I never got there! Knowlsey came rushing in.

"Pack up, Sal, we leave in an hour! We're going to the Philippine Islands!"

Love, Sally B.

I remember —

Another unfinished night duty — my second! Once again we packed footlockers, suitcases and my beloved pail now full of shoes. I hoped I could take my bureau-desk Val had made me and I did. So we donned our helmets, gas mask cases, backpacks, and canteens and were loaded into trucks to go to Humboldt Bay where we had landed in September.

We hardly had time to say good-bye to the friends we had made here at the 51st who were permanently assigned. They had been so friendly and helpful. I could not even say good-bye to the wonderful ward men whose service had been so essential and effective. I did run in to say good-bye to the patients who had just come in from the Philippines where I would be going.

We just pulled up stakes and left, riding one last time through the deep rain forest, on the wonderful road built by our Seabees. Over the red earth, past the smiling native people, down to the sea where landing craft waited to transport us to a white hospital ship, the *Emily H. M. Weder*, anchored way out in the harbor. Stage two had begun. This was December 26th, 1944.

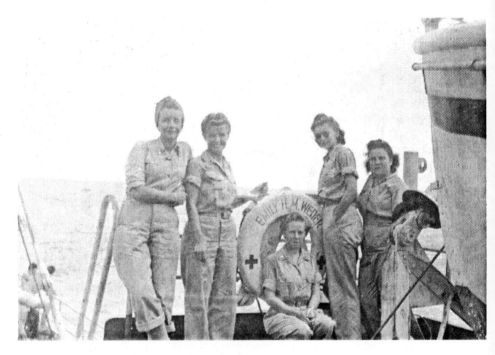

Above: BC, me, Knowlsey, Shirl and Mickey on board the *Emily H. M. Weder.*

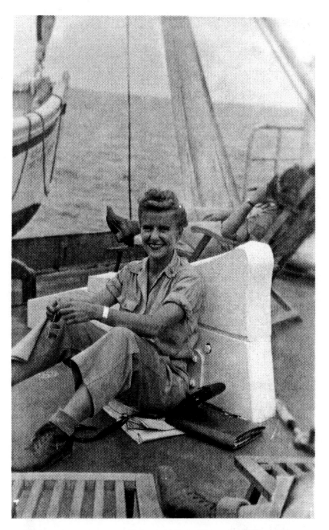

Writing a letter home from aboard the *Emily
H. M. Weder.*

CHAPTER FOUR

At Sea, the *Emily H. M. Weder*

December 30, 1944

Dear Mom and Dad,

… We're on shipboard still in the harbor. We've been watching the activity going on onshore in the harbor and in the air. It's a beautiful tropical spot — coral reefs, lovely graceful beaches with overhanging palms. All we can see are these lovely spots with the huge mountains behind. It is a strange feeling to me to have lived here, been part of this spot and to know I'll never see it again. I'm sure it will never be the same in the future as it is now.

We've had a wonderful time on board seeing all our old casual group who were not sent with the four of us to the 51st. We had much to share. When we don't write letters or read, we play bridge. In the evening we sit on deck, on chairs under this starry sky with the moon shining. Sometimes we see a movie. Sounds tough, doesn't it?

The other day I got to talking with an MP. He wanted some Dutch currency in which we are paid here. So, I gave him some. Won't be able to use guilders in the Philippines. He couldn't make change but that night he gave the five of us iced Cokes, real American Cokes!! They were so good. Tonight he gave me a crisp, fresh apple!!

The other morning a group of us were harmonizing when the ship's doctor begged us to sing over the ship's loud speaker. We did. We called ourselves the "Joy Girls of Radio, Hello, Hello, Hello!" For that little deed we got more Cokes. They are a most hospitable group on this ship, which was the one that brought all the men to me on Christmas Eve!!

How pleasant it is to sit here, cool, no bugs, good food. Don't worry if you don't hear for a while. I'll write as soon as I can. Good-bye New Guinea!!! Good-bye Hollandia!!

Love, Me

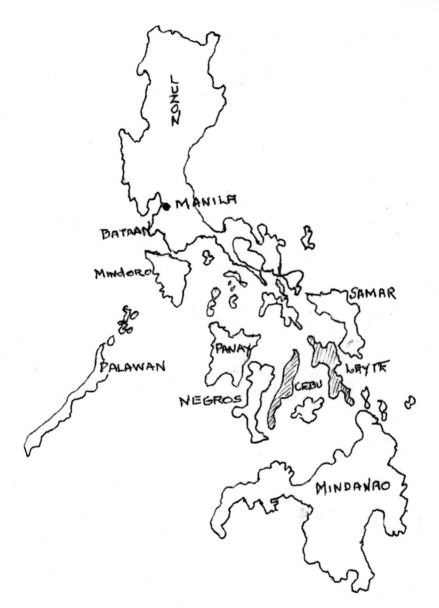

Map of the Philippine Islands - Darkened areas are islands I visited.

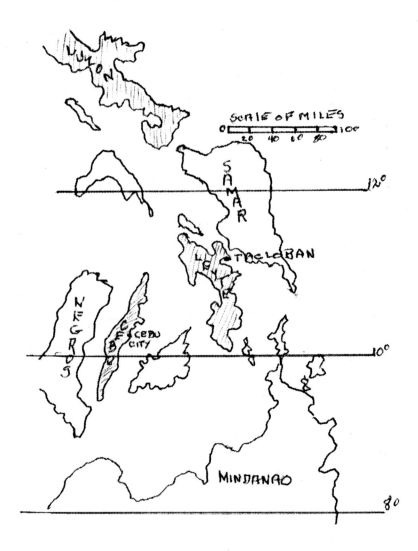

Location of Leyte and Cebu in relation to other Philippine Islands.

CHAPTER FIVE

The Philippines

January 3, 1945

Dear Mom and Dad,

… We're here!! During our trip up I was face down in my bunk with hot packs to my fanny because of a crop of boils, uncomfortable but all too common to many of us in these tropics. The Doc lanced mine, hence the packs! But it's taken about three days to get here.

We've been maneuvering around islands all day, lovely green ones, rising abruptly out of the ocean and disappearing just as fast on the other side. We are anchored way out in a harbor. (*Tacloban Harbor in Leyte.*)

Two Filipino children came along side in their outrigger canoe. The sail was deep tan with bright yellow patches. The kids were so cheery and greeted us in English. The little girl wore a beige dress. She stood in the bow with a coolie hat in her hand that she traded to a sergeant for his shirt! Her brother was a charming little boy who had a brilliant white smile in his brown face. He wore a yellow straw hat, turned up at the front, a burlap shirt and very blue pants. He traded his hat for a sailor hat.

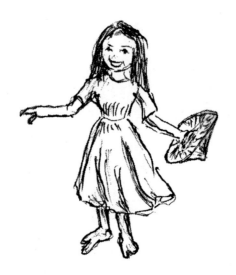

Little sister in the outrigger's bow.

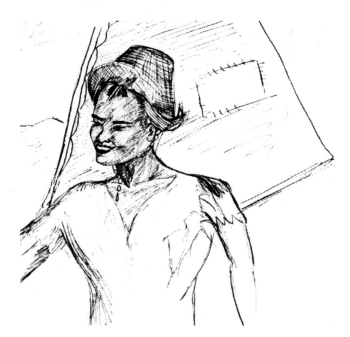

The boy in the outrigger.

I ran down to the open hold to snap a picture before an MP chased me out. The kids hung around all afternoon trading for shells and coins. Such a picture they made against the blue-green sea and the green hills behind. It's hard to believe there is still so much activity going on here. But here we are out at sea, waiting. The trip has been a good chance to rest to prepare for what's coming. This is what we were sent over to do, to care for our men in the Battle of the Philippines! And we're finally moving into anchor. It's getting dark so maybe tomorrow we'll hit the beach!

Love, Sally B.

Leyte

I recall —

The Philippine Islands are made up of thousands of islands, from tiny ones to huge ones like Mindanao. Leyte is located at about the middle of the north-south line but on the eastern edge of the archipelago. Samar hugs Leyte's northeast corner and Luzon, home to Manila, is due north.

Leyte was one of the more underdeveloped islands. It was rural in character, home to farmers who raised rice, sugar cane, coconuts and hemp, and many men who fished locally in their outriggers. We saw very few cars. Most goods were transported by a two-wheeled wagon hitched to a patient carabao (water buffalo). Roads were greatly improved by the Army, but gravel surfaced.

The people were warm and friendly, eager to relate to those of us who were there in the Army. Close family ties existed. The Catholic Church was dominant and the churches in the villages were the largest and loveliest buildings. Many Spanish cultural patterns persist as does their Spanish currency.

Recreation was family and village-centered. There were village dances. The whole family, from 90 years to nine months went. The young girls wore cotton, western clothes and their black hair was often permed. The older women usually wore long black tube skirts with either a simple cotton blouse or, for festivals, beautiful, sheer pina cloth puff-sleeved blouses. Their hair was usually pulled back into a bun. The women's footgear was clogs, carved sandals or bare feet. I cannot recall ever seeing a woman in shorts or pants.

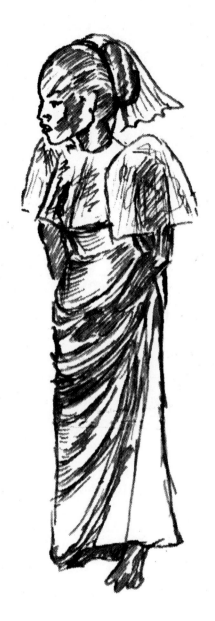

A Philippine woman

Family homes in the country were simple. A small square structure on stilts, thatched with woven bamboo sides and entered by a ladder, seemed to be the usual village home. Sanitation was crude. Animals — pigs, carabao and chickens, ran around under the houses. Gardens were planted in the yard.

Washing hung in the sun. It was often done by rubbing it on stones at the edge of the river and then rinsing it there. Because of poor sanitation, parasitic infestations were common, often more than one type.

Men farmed or fished. For fun, there were cockfights, a big weekend activity. Long elaborate metal spurs, sharp and deadly were fastened to the cocks' legs. Many spurs were family heirlooms and very valuable. It was the hope that one cock would cut the other to ribbons. It was so cruel!

Education had been on hold when we arrived, but schools did open. English was taught in the schools. It was nice to be able to converse and relate to these friendly people in an understandable way.

Leyte, what I saw of it on the eastern seaboard primarily and during one foray across the mountains to Carigara on the north, was a lovely spot. Ten degrees above the Equator, it was hot and humid with a monsoon-like climate. Its black beaches were beautiful and living on the beach, as we did at the end, was perfect.

Wild animal life was rare. We saw birds, egrets I believe. We saw a monitor lizard, geckos by the thousand, tarantulas and scorpions. I'm sure snakes existed but had long hidden from the activity of our hospital.

Flora was different from Hollandia. There were many palms and other large-leafed trees grew there too. Flowers and grasses covered all open land. Much of the land was under cultivation. Coconut palms were everywhere.

I'm sure now Leyte is no longer a backward island. It became a bustling port during our stay. I'm sure its capital, Tacloban, is no longer a dirt-streeted town.

The help given to us by the Filipino people, both men and women, lessened the strain on all of us who were so shorthanded. They were eager to help, and were warm and willing partners. The title the Filipinos all used for the nurses was "Mum" (for "Mam"). When agreeing to do a task, they always said, "I will be the one, Mum." It was an unforgettable phrase.

January through March
We Land

January 4, 1945

Dear Mom and Dad,

Right after I mailed your letter from the ship last night, we were told to be ready to debark at once. Off we went to pack up. My gear was ready. I slung on the musette bag, canteen and first aid pack on my pistol belt. My gas mask was on my right shoulder, pocketbook over my left and my field coat strapped to my back. My helmet was on my head. "Hurry up and wait" was our Army slogan! So, we waited a long while to get off — until it was very dark. When the time came, I held my precious pail, now full of shoes, in my left hand, my suitcase in my right and went down the gangplank into a landing barge. We were crowded, but off we went to shore.

It was a thrill to land on Philippine soil on a very narrow, dark beach about seven feet wide. No one was there to meet us. On a dune or beach bank was a tangle of barbed wire. It was 10 p.m., January 3, 1945. We lighted our cigarettes, began to sing, hoping someone would come for us. No one. We sat all alone for about a half-hour, then a firm muffled voice yelled, "Who's there?"

We looked into the barrels of several guns.

"We're nurses for the 126th General!"

"Never heard of it!"

"We were just landed from a hospital ship. We're waiting to be met!"

"What the hell. Don't you know there's a war on? Your voices carry across water to the Nips. We have six to eight raids a night! For God's sake, put out your cigarettes and shut up!"

That was our introduction to the Philippines!

Oh, well, our two charge lieutenants arranged for us to move through the wire into the camp of some engineers.

Once we were in this area, the engineers made us hot coffee and turkey sandwiches, and we had real pickles. It all tasted wonderful, but they were plenty upset about the way we had been dumped ashore.

About midnight, three trucks came for us. We loaded bag and baggage and began our drive through the mud. The GIs gave us such a cheery welcome. "Welcome, gals!" Many whistles and shouts and we were on our way somewhere. The truck lights were hooded so we went slowly through a big town and some small ones. We saw old Spanish churches that had been shelled, real houses with metal filigree decorations — but bombed or shelled. We were singing and laughing. By 2 a.m., we arrived somewhere in a grove of coconut palms and much mud, but not our 126th General, which was not yet finished.

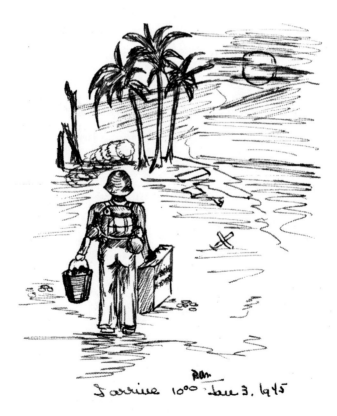

I arrive January 3, 1945

The outfit where we were put down, we learned, was the 133rd General. On the spur of the moment they erected a tent and filled it with canvas cots. We gathered up our gear, crossed a bridge and plunked down onto a cot. One happy GI told me not to fall into the water because there were crocodiles! Maybe yes, maybe no. I never saw one (*but, months later, I saw a monitor lizard*).

There were no mosquito nets. I used some of my canteen water in my helmet to wash in, hung the full helmet on my cot, slathered repellent all over my face and hands, pulled on an extra coat and fell asleep in my clothes. We were cold.

Early the next morning someone called "Air Raid! Zeros overhead!" Quickly we rolled out of bed and under our cots jamming our helmets on as we went. Mine was still full of last night's wash water! I got a good drenching. There were bombs and there was a fire. We learned that the air strip was nearby in Tanauan and the Corsairs were constantly up, five up and five down so's not to lose all the planes at once and to protect the air strip. We were all scared.

We learned that Zeros do not sound like our smoothly humming planes. Zeros sound like washing machines. Soon we could recognize them by sound. We've had many blackouts at night and in the morning for a while.

This was my first night on Leyte. Early, but after the air raid, we sloshed to chow, a memorable breakfast for me! I sat opposite a 1st lieutenant, a patient whose hand was encompassed in a huge bandage.

"Hi, where did you come from?" he asked, his eyes twinkling. "We arrived last night from New Guinea." I answered. "Like bridge?" he asked. "Sure do," I said. "Name's Dan," he said. I told him mine.

All around us native people were building with bamboo and thatching. Women were sitting and weaving palm fronds together to make a section of a Nipa roof. We saw some women pounding clothes on stones in the brook. An old gentleman in a large hat, Julian by name, urged us to visit his village next door where people of all ages seemed glad to see us. He put a baby puppy in each of our arms. Activity was everywhere, hens, roosters, pigs, dogs and children all running around.

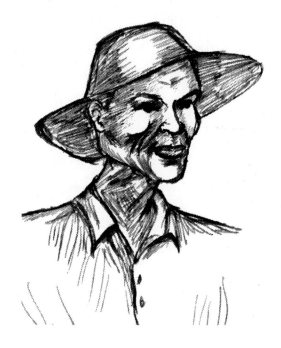

Julian

When we returned to our tents, there were many children all around speaking English. I shouldn't have been surprised, but I was. After all, the Philippines had been a Territory since 1898. One question I asked that first morning was about speaking English. Our young woman Nipa-roof builder told us that there were hundreds of Philippine Islands all speaking different dialects. English was taught in all the schools, nonfunctional since the Japanese invasion, but it was a unifying language. The other language spoken was Tagolag, a universal Filipino language which all island residents could use with each other and get by, since each island had its own dialect. This was very interesting to me.

Three shy little girls began to sing "My native land, my native land" to the tune of "My Maryland." They showed us a plant they called, Har-u-pa-i (sensitive plant). When you touch the top leaves they collapse, touching the branches below and they collapse, and so on all the way down until there is only a stick!! (I never got over the fun of making a plant collapse and watching it become a leafed plant again!)

Later in the morning, we met a bright 17-year-old girl, Christine, who had been in high school when the Nips came. She hoped to go back to finish, then go to the university to train to be a teacher.

We asked her about the Japs. "We don't like them. They kill without sin."

"What did you do when they were here?"

"I stayed in my house, so I won't be molested."

"Do you want to get married?"

"Oh no, times are too unsettled!"

She added that the GIs try to teach them how to Jitterbug but added, "It's too hard, but we're glad they're here."

I've been here 16 hours! We'll be helping at the 133rd here until the 126th is done. It's a good place, muddy, friendly, and busy. I'm here ready to GO!

What a tragedy about Jeremy Graves! I can't believe he's gone. How sad!! And so close to coming home. And how relieved I am to know brother John is still home and safe. How wonderful for you both not to have to worry anymore about our flyer!!

So glad you have Mr. Duff (a Scottish Terrier). He'll be lots of fun to walk with!!

Love, Me

Detached Service
133rd General Hospital

January 10, 1945

Dear Mom and Dad,

We've been here a week, a wonderful one despite the rain and the mud! OH, what mud — and all the inconveniences where women are not expected!!

I'm working seven hours a day on a surgical ward. There are two of us for ten patients. Not hard. During my off hours, I've been squired around by Dan, the young officer I met that first breakfast.

He and his four companions, all of the 7th Infantry Division, have adopted the five of us and we've had a lot of sightseeing.

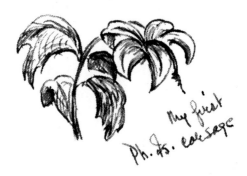

My first Philippine corsage.

One afternoon they took us to see our neighborhood! We went to a native town then out to the airstrip. We stopped to pick a hibiscus blossom of bright red, like the ones in New Guinea. At the airstrip we saw many different kinds of planes. The men helped us identify a few. There are piles of wrecked Zeros along the edges. A Filipino man asked Dan for a cigarette and he gave him one. The old man shrewdly turned it once in his grimy hand and popped paper and all into his mouth, gave one long sigh of satisfaction and turned on his heel. "Making a plug out of a Camel! How about that!" Dan was laughing, "No accounting for tastes!!"

In the evening the group plays bridge, or we sketch or write letters. Our leisure facilities are pretty limited. We have a "Rec" tent, but we sit on boxes or logs and play bridge on a box. There is a light bulb overhead, the company is fun and we enjoy the diversion.

Yesterday, in the rain we went to the village to see the cathedral. The inside of it was lovely. There were high vaulted ceilings, painted walls with only a few bomb or shell scars. This was used as a field hospital[9] when our troops first arrived.

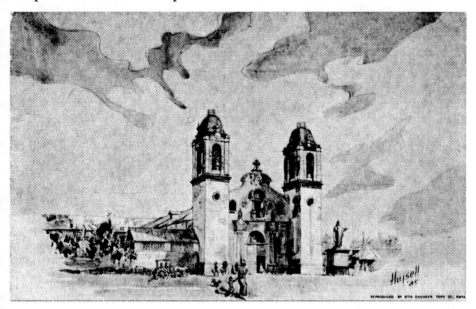

The Cathedral in Palo, Leyte.

In the town, we saw water buffalo (carabao), the beast of burden here, rice paddies and people of all ages from eighty to six months. We visited a school, closed for three years. It had been opened only three weeks ago. We talked to the principal who told us where his stacks of books had been hidden for three years. On our way back to the jeep, I stepped in a huge mud hole, the gooiest, stickiest mud I've ever seen. The group all stood laughing. Dan with his hands on his hips, his legs astride, arms akimbo — laughing. Oh well, back at the hospital I stood under a faucet and washed my whole right side, pants, socks and shoes. Tomorrow these guys report down the coast to their outfit. Too bad! They were lots of fun.

[9] This hospital in the Cathedral at Palo was written up and photographed for the December 25, 1944 edition of "Life" magazine.

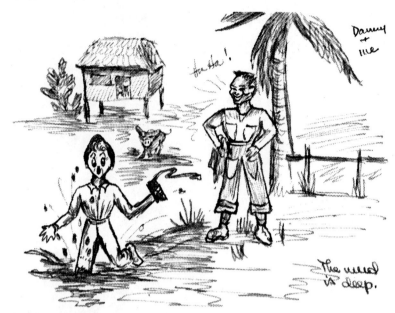

I fell in the mud the afternoon Dan took us to town.

We're now sitting in our tent ward on typhoon alert. Everything is anchored down. We're here with two days of personal supplies, helmets and musette bags, ready to stay indefinitely. It may not come, but if it does, we're ready. Hope I'm not hit by a flying coconut!

It's great to be here, my big adventure and one I'll never forget. Working hard makes the time fly.

All of a sudden, my friend Dan has appeared, flung himself on an empty bed and is drawing! He does not belong on this enlisted men's ward. The guys wonder about him — It's nice for me to have a "guardian angel."

Love, Sally B.

The 126th General Hospital Opens

January 15, 1945

Dear Folks,

... Oh, how it's rained, but no typhoon, just mud all over the boards, which serve as paths and now sink when you walk. You run over the boards before they have time to sink out of sight. It's quite an experience, this rain and mud!! No injuries. But the Big News is on January 13th, we came to our own 126th General! We're where we belong at last!!

Love, Me

History of the 126th General

A small diversion about the history of the 126th General reprinted from the anniversary issue of the *"Sauna News."*[10]

"SAUNA NEWS"

Friday, 21 September 1945 **Vol. 1. No. 235**

"San Francisco, September 21, 1944 ... on this date the *S.S. Monterey* carried the 126th General Hospital to overseas service. Her holds were laden with tons of equipment needed to establish a modern Army hospital under tropical conditions. The huge liner

---

[10] "Sauna News" was the regular publication put out by the 126th General Hospital in Palo, Leyte in 1945.

steamed down the Bay as dozens of grateful Americans cheered it along.

… Consisting of 441 enlisted men, 54 officers, 5 dietitians and physiotherapists and 5 Red Cross workers, all had come from Harmon General at Longview, Texas to Camp Stoneman.

Known as the 'duty-doingest outfit' ever to stage at Stoneman, the 126th put its training to good use on board the *Monterey* with its men on almost every conceivable detail. Some played in the band for tea dances … There were 900 WACs aboard during the crossing and Major Nathan Kohan, their executive officer, was drafted into serving as a baby in King Neptune's Court during the traditional ceremonies at the Equator. [11]

… Finally, boarded on the *HMAS Manoora*, an Australian Troop ship, for transport to the east coast of Leyte Island in the Philippines Archipelago, the first section headed north. The 300 remaining tons unable to be loaded on the *Manoora* were put on the *SS George G. Meade* … And on the *Manoora*, in the middle of a flock of poker games and one good bridge game, the convoy's radar picked up unidentified aircraft, and on November 13, the morning report carried a note: 'Attacked by enemy aircraft at 1630: No casualties.' Below decks, the men heard over the PA system the details of the battle, in which the lone plane which came into the convoy was shot down.

On the following day the outfit landed at Red Beach near Palo, Leyte. As the first landing wave went over the sides of the ship onto

---

[11] These personnel were landed to stage as we were, in Hollandia on October 10, 1944, a month after we had arrived.

the landing nets, a Jap Betty came in to attack and strafe. Leonard Clawson, sitting in an ambulance hanging on a crane over the ship's hold, swore he was about to jump when ack-ack got the attacker. Men on deck watched in awe as a P-38 over the beach caught and shot down another plane. Again, the morning report read: 'No casualties.'

By 1800 on November 14, the male section of the detachment, 50 officers, 441 enlisted men, a warrant officer had moved to the organizational area, 3 kilometers west of Palo on the banks of the Palo River.

There they found MUD, rotten coconuts, and there they labored long and arduously, first to drain the area, then to build the installation.

… The site was a morass of mud littered with rotten coconut hulls and topped by palms that were almost jungle-thick. The 126thers slopped hip deep through mud to find a place to put up shelter halves so they could rest before tackling the job ahead of them.

There was no passage for vehicles beyond the main road to Palo. There was no bridge over the Palo River for several weeks, only a footpath. Water stood feet deep in spots all over the site.

Wallowing along the bank up the river, men set up the present detachment area first, then with fingers crossed, set out to see what could be done. At one time, the engineers assigned to the project said it wasn't any use, but the work went on. Nobody could count the times the 126thers said the same thing, but the work went on.

Before General Kirk could reach Leyte, they'd reclaimed 50 acres of seemingly impossible mud holes, unsuited even for foxholes, or so it looked. They'd drained the swamps and filled the roadbeds on a corduroy base of coconut logs covered with gravel to extend 2.3 miles of road over what has seemed like quicksand. They had put up canvas for 64 squad tents in the detachment area and more than 30 ward tents and an uncountable number of tents in the officers' and nurses' area, enough canvas to cover Washington Square in New York; enough canvas to roof over one tenth of Vatican City.

They put up frames too, to hold that 373,712 square feet of canvas and they had to put board flooring under every tent. They built offices and supply rooms, and a chapel of bamboo. They had constructed in a forgotten Palo coconut grove, a hospital with more beds than there were in the whole state of Nevada in the year 1943.

They'd used 255,000 board feet of lumber putting in 170,000 feet of one inch, 55,000 feet of 2x4s and an additional 30,000 feet of larger stuff.

They'd set up a water system, capable of handling 100,000 gallons of water a day, a generator system which could light the city of Macomb, Illinois, and steam plants, an incinerator and a laundry unit giving far quicker service than the poor civilians got back home. They engineered this grove into a hustling city of 3,500!

... The months from our opening, January 13, to April were incredible. On January 15 when the original patient registry was opened, 15 men were admitted. There were 206 the next day and an additional 300 beds were available and soon to be filled. By January 29, the patient load was 1,034.

On February 15, the first Japanese POW's were admitted to the stockade wards. Two months and 12 days after our hospital opened, patient number 10,000 was admitted on March 12th. On June 5, patient number 20,000 was admitted. Hundreds of patients went through the Convalescent Training Program."[12]

January 15, 1945

Dear Folks,

... So here we are finally at the 126th!! It's a lovely spot next to the rice fields with the patient carabao rising and falling in and out of mud holes. There are lovely white birds like the egrets I drew in New Guinea. They perch on the treetops and look like huge snow drifts. Suddenly they move and the tree is summer again! There are only six of us in this large tent with a wooden floor so we each have plenty of room.

Love, Me

January 18, 1945

Dear Mom and Dad,

The nurses' quarters are off to the far end. There are six of us in each tent. We each have an iron bed, T-bars with netting, a pillow,

[12] "Sauna News", Vol I #235, September 1945, p. 5, 6

sheets and a pillowcase, towels and a space about five by seven feet. Whatever the dimensions, it does not seem crowded.

Our tents are on wooden platforms and we are all interconnected by raised wooden-slatted walks leading to the showers, the john (holes in wood again) in an enclosed structure. There is a washing room with actual machines in which we can wash our clothes. Eventually, we may have young Filipino girls come to wash and iron our pants and shirts. Up to now we have washed, hung our shirts on hangers, and put the trousers under our mattress to give a semblance of press!

This whole area is separate from the main activities in this huge unit. It is relatively quiet, convenient. The palm trees cover our tents so we have shade. We also have Geckos, small harmless lizards that run nimbly in the support system of all the tents, eating insects and talking saying, "Gecko-Gecko." They have special hooks on their feet so they can climb anywhere!

Our quarters are across the lane from the Women's Ward, then comes the mess hall. Off to the side of the nurses' area is the night nurses' sleeping quarters. A Nipa-thatched, screened building is for those of us who work the twelve hours (7 p.m. to 7 a.m.) night shift. We were glad to be apart from the hospital bustle in a Nipa-thatched building which is the best that could be offered to let us sleep in as cool a place as possible. (It is NOT cool.) It is hot and sleep is restless and sweaty, but there was an attempt to make the day sleep of the night nurses as comfortable as possible. So here we are. We settled in that first day. Then Captain McKay called us all together and told us we would have patients in 48 hours. We must order linen, drugs, make up beds and be ready to receive a full contingent of patients. I can't wait to be assigned to help. Captain McKay is our Chief Nurse. She's regular Army and quite demanding. She escaped from Luzon when the Japanese came.

Love, Sally B.

First Head Nurse Assignment — Ward #16

I remember —

"Lt. Hitchcock, you will be in charge of Ward #16!" I was amazed! I was to be in charge of getting one new unit ready. It was my baby! So with the lists in hand, I flew off to find this place. I had a map in my hand and I walked, then ran on and on. Near the far end of the hospital was my ward. On it were two wonderful ward men to be with me for many months, Sgts. Bannister and Bruno.

Sgt. Bruno was tall, strong, dark and graying at the temples. He was between 40 and 45 I'd guess — always quiet, helpful, ready to do more than his fair share. Bannister was a tall, curly-haired, rosy-faced blond in his twenties, but under the strong, quiet leadership of Bruno, he became the same kind of wonderful team player.

We began. I had a unit of 60 beds: 30 on one side, 30 on the other side of the nursing station, which is in the middle. We called for crates of linen, two sheets per bed, and extras, pillow cases, beds, mattresses, pillows, wash clothes, towels, glasses, pitchers, bath blankets, T-bars, mosquito nets, soap, toothpaste, brushes, pajama tops and bottoms, bedside stands, wash basins, emesis basins, soap dishes, and drugs, narcotics, sedatives, analgesics, atabrine, penicillin, specimen cups, lab slips, pen, ink, and all the chart forms we'd need.

Fifty-odd years later, I remember the plan Miss McKay made for each linen cupboard and each drug cupboard. Everything was to be in exactly the same spot on every unit. And was that a help! When we moved around, we never had to look far for anything. It was always in the same place. We fussed at first, but were grateful in the very near future!

So, the orders went in and trucks arrived with our supplies. What a scramble! Up went the beds, mattresses, T-bars, mosquito netting. We washed beds, we made beds. Then came the bedside units, bowls, basins, soap, urinals, bedpans, linen and a newspaper trash envelope at exactly the same spot on each bed!

Soon the beds were done. Some Filipino men were helping to open boxes and carry supplies. It was at this point where we, who were grateful for a bully-beef sandwich, discovered that to work for us they wanted rice, NOT bully beef. "If the Japanese gave rice, why not you?" they would ask. This was something to ponder. We kept on working. This was an administrative problem, not mine, but it made me think! Food seemed to be so much more important than politics!!

That first day Bruno, Bannister and I worked from 7 a.m. to 2 a.m. the next morning. We dropped for a few hours and came back at 7 a.m. It was really taking shape. When the first patients began to arrive that afternoon from Luzon (the invasion began January 9), we were ready and waiting. By night, we had 42 patients — no acutely ill men, but we had dysenteries, malarias, some wounds, skin diseases, sick medical problems. There was a lot to do to make charts, name tags and bed tags for all these men and get to know them!! I began 6:30 a.m. rounds the next morning.

January 21, 1945

Dear Mom and Dad,

To get to know all my patients and their problems, I planned to do what we had been taught to do at Yale, go to work early and make rounds before the doctors came. So having a quick breakfast, I went off to #16. With my notebook in hand, I went up and down the wards, speaking to each patient and listening to his complaints. By the time the doctor came, I had quite a list.

At first, the doctor went with me as together we made rounds. But then a few days later, when he came he began to ask for my notes from which he wrote patient orders. This was very upsetting to me. The patients wanted to discuss their problems with the doctor.

I know I'm griping, but — we are not hitting it off at all!!

Love, Me

January 26, 1945

Dear Folks,

… So it's been long hours, 14 straight, and we are told to expect 12-14 hour days from now on. There is a lot of fighting going on islands around us so we have many patients.

My main goal has been to do well with my first head nurse assignment, to take the best care of my patients and run a shipshape ward. Shirl is head nurse on Isolation and doing well. BC and Mickey are on nights and Knowlsey is slaving on days so we don't connect too often. You can see why I don't get to write too many letters. I owe everyone.

I have to add before I close that we still have a lot of air activity. It's disconcerting because at night when we try to play bridge, or see a movie, we have a blackout almost nightly. We can't sit in a movie without a blackout-flash of three flares, red in the sky, then a blackout. No cigarettes, no nothing. Then the all clear, two red flares and the movie goes back on.

When we get up in the morning at 0600 the early morning blackout comes and we have to dress and comb our hair in the dark. It's a challenge and an inconvenience. Our hospital is not a target, for which we are grateful.

Oh, and all the nurses have had to give up their beds in exchange for canvas cots again. Our patient load is so great the guys who are sick get the beds. We're all used to the cots. We had them for months in New Guinea.

Love, Me

February 3, 1945

Dear Mom and Dad,

… Whew, I've been given four wards with 40 patients each. We are so short of help and have so many hurt men. It is a 12-14 hour grind or more. Needless to say, we are terribly busy. When I get off at night and try to write letters, there's a blackout.

Now my ward officer and I are not doing well at all. I feel badly for the patients and for me. It's a brand new feeling to want to fight with this man — and he outranks me!!

… His lack of concern and diagnostic testing upsets me. One such case was a man who complained of abdominal pain and was discharged as a goldbrick.[13]

No diagnostic tests were done!! He was soon readmitted and he was found to be positive for amoebic dysentery — and he worked in our kitchen!

Another case, and I record these because I came in open conflict with this MD, was a young man admitted with severe lower-right-side abdominal pain.

The only orders I found were to "purge" him (giving a severe cathartic to look for parasites) and send a "sample." The doctor had done no physical exam and no blood work before this treatment. So, I asked him if he did not want to write further orders after the physical exam. He told me to follow his orders!

I was shocked, and told him I refused to purge the patient until the physical and blood work was done. I had done an abdominal exam and found this lad's abdomen was rigid and had rebound tenderness and he had right lower-quadrant pain. This was not my

---

[13] Goldbrick — a term commonly used to refer to someone who avoids work by faking a problem.

job but I told the doctor what I found. He was furious and stalked off telling me to do what I wanted!

I called the lab for an emergency CBC (complete blood count). It was done. The count came back along with the Chief of Surgery. The white count was 40,000. The lad was rushed to surgery where a red-hot appendix was removed. The Chief of Surgery did not scold me; he praised me. My ward officer was speechless with fury.

This problem continued. When this man became really abusive in his language and openly critical and sarcastic about the way I had questioned one of his orders for a patient, I felt he had become unprofessional and in my own mind, incompetent.

After a lot of thought I screwed up my courage and went to my chief nurse to ask her to change my assignment. She asked a lot of questions that I tried to answer fairly. She finally got me to tell her all my concerns. I was very upset. She was entirely non-committal.

The next day on the ward when I met the doctor, he asked me who had reported him.

"I did," I replied.

"Why," he asked. I don't know how I dared to say what I did, but I answered.

"Sir, can you honestly say to yourself that you are giving these men the best care they deserve?"

To my surprise, I was not moved. He was.

To climax all this "to do," Captain McKay told me I was to be head nurse on the Women's Ward.

"We want someone with strength of her own convictions, so we have chosen you!" she told me. So, I'll move again. I feel this is a huge challenge, to be relatively untried as a new graduate (old as I am) and in charge of a big women's ward of my peers!

Love, Sally B.

Second Head Nurse Assignment
Women's Ward #25

February 6, 1945

Dear Folks,

… How I wish we'd get some more nurses. We are all so very tired, but I have to say, this unit is friendly and all of us work very hard. I'll keep you posted, but I probably won't write so often. I wanted to serve and I'm doing it. We all are and we are really helping so many.

… How I miss Bruno and Bannister and my patients on Ward #16. It had all become so familiar. The young Filipino girls who helped were so willing.

Now I really am challenged! I have all services, medical, surgical, GYN, and neuro-psychiatric and all the various physicians who care for all these problems. It is confusing and challenging to have all those services, to keep all the orders straight and to always get the right patient with the right doctor. But familiarity helps. This is the main women's ward for Base K.

Surprise. I went out one night with a Navy man I knew in Hollandia. He is from Connecticut. He took me to a nearby village, a citizen's village, where we shopped at "shops!" I bought my first item in the Philippines, an abaca (hemp) table cloth. There were counters of dried fish, pottery jars.

Children were milling around. The little ones wear no pants, just long shirts. One little girl asked me my name and I told her "Sally." How she laughed, "Sol-ly" she repeated. Guess it's weird to them not to have names they are used to. Then he took me to a cockfight. Never again!!! It was gruesome. The men put knives on the cock's legs and watch and cheer as these birds slice each other up!!

Love Sally B.

I remember —

Early in February, American POWs were freed during the Luzon liberation and brought to the 126th. This was when the women from Santo Tomas came to me on Ward 25 and General Wainright was admitted to a men's floor.

The prisoners taken at Bataan and incarcerated for the duration in Santo Tomas University in Manila on Luzon were finally liberated. General Jonathan Wainwright had remained to command the American and Filipino forces on the peninsula of Bataan and the island of Corregidor. He was forced to surrender in April of 1942. Along with his troops who survived the brutal march and any other allied personnel including the nurses and doctors, he became a prisoner of war for three years. Slowly and systematically, the Japanese cut daily calories to about 750, so that when Santo Tomas was liberated in February 1945, the general and other POWs were almost too weak to stand.

Nurses from Santo Tomas

February 13, 1945

Dear Mom and Dad,

It's been an amazing week! The nurses liberated from Manila in Luzon came to my floor. They had been kept as POWs at Santo Tomas University. They said they had not had any medicine and they systematically were being starved by the Japanese, but had not been physically abused. We had to check them over for serious problems before they are sent home. Aside from being very thin, they do not seem to be chronically ill.

When we learned they were coming, all our women collected deodorant, lipstick, toothpaste and powder — anything we had from home that we could give to them as a little something to cheer them on their way.

They were so appreciative and uncomplaining. We were thrilled to be able to do something, small as it is, for these brave women who had been incarcerated so long. They are brave! We are all humbled by their courage and their fortitude.

I can't tell you anymore. We've been asked not to repeat what they say for security reasons.

Mom and Dad, one of the nurses, Mary Reppack, lives in Connecticut. She will take some of my treasures home and get the Red Cross to mail them to you.

Something else wonderful happened to me the other night. I saw a "Christmas tree"! I couldn't believe my eyes. There were millions of tiny lights all through a palm tree. Fireflies. Dan had told me about seeing a tree like this, this past Christmas Eve on Leyte, his fourth away from home. Leyte was his fourth Christmas away and Leyte was his fourth campaign. Attu and Kiska (the Aleutian Islands), Kwajalein (Marshall Islands) and Leyte. That tree was memorable.

I guess you know where I am now. I'm 10 miles from the town you mentioned.

And the other wonderful event was that I asked Captain McKay if it would be possible for me to get Bruno and Bannister transferred from Ward #16 to my Women's Ward. And they were transferred! They arrived all smiles. I'm so happy. We are a good team.

Love, Sally B.

February 23, 1945

Dear Mom and Dad,

… The work goes on. It is hard but interesting. The other night two of Dan's pals came up and BC and I played some high powered bridge. It's good to stay put because it is hard to drive blacked out at night in the mud on the narrow roads. So, we had a killer game. These two men are such good friends.

Thanks, you two, for your Valentines. I loved them. 'Twas lovely. Got one from Dan, who was sent to Biak for health reasons. It said —

> "I'd much prefer to be drinking beer
>
> But since I haven't any and chances are
>
> damn slight I'd get any for quite a
>
> while, how's about your being my
>
> Valentine, Dear?"

Silly!

Annie's still in Hawaii. Both Selma and Spraguey are in France. We Yalie's will have much to share!

Love, Me

February 28, 1945

Dear Folks,

… I'm back at work again. Boils be damned. Major Heath said if I was admitted for this boil problem again, he'd evacuate me! Fat chance I'll turn in again. I don't want to go home. My pals need every pair of hands there are!! Anyway, I'm not the only one. Many gals and guys have this problem. It's the heat and dripping clothes all the time.

Went out with June and her friend, a Marine from Hollandia and his friend. They took us to a native dance. It was in a school building and all ages, ninety to nine months were there. We were the only nurses. We danced to their music and met the mayor of the village. My date told the orchestra leader my name was Sally. Promptly the band played, "I Wonder What's Become of Sally." I was told to turn around, then a young woman nudged me, "For you, Mum!" as she hummed the tune. They always call us "Mum."

One night, Don, a buddy of Dan's came to visit us. He's such a nice young man who is 28 and he admits he's scared. He's been through all major campaigns with Dan and ER. Only ten of his original group are left. He says his chances of coming back are only one in 50. Don asked me the other night if I believed in God. "Of course I do," I answered.

"Please pray for us all then," he said. It was so sad to realize how terrible his next few weeks were to be!! I feel so humble before these guys and honored to be their friend!! We are all praying for them. They are so exceptionally fine. *(And he did come back alive!)*

Love, Me

March 2, 1945

Dear Dad,

A birthday letter for you for the 22nd so I'll be sure you get it. Have a wonderful year, Dad. A momentous year for you, Dad, the first year of retirement, but you and Mom seem to be filling each day so full and having fun in your new town and new state of Vermont. Do you miss Connecticut, your home for thirty-three years?

I'd love to be home to celebrate your day, but I'm only 17,537 miles away. Hey, it's closer than New Guinea!

Remember how we used to walk to my school together on your way to work, trying to keep *out of step* with each other and laughing and being foolish? We had a lot of fun. I'll always remember those walks to school. And the friends who joined us and laughed and laughed, who thought it was wonderful to laugh and be foolish with my Dad! Lots to remember.

And Dad, I feel I am so lucky having a Pop like you!! Have a very Happy Birthday. And please take $10.00 out of my bank account and buy something you want, some shrubs, a book, something you really want for yourself.

With love from me!!!

March 9, 1945

Dear Folks,

… What a lovely evening. The men are playing baseball on our new field across the road and their yells sound so like home.

Last Tuesday Dan and his friends, the ones we all like so much, came for one last fling before they are shipped out. We all went down to one of the pillboxes by the beach (*at Tacloban Harbor*) and sang and talked. We were popping corn over a fire. We had some beer and sandwiches. It was so cozy.

Suddenly they threw sand on the fire and yelled, "GET INTO THE PILL BOX!" We did in a hurry, then we heard it. A lone Jap plane came in low, dropped bombs on the big fuel dump by the harbor. Feeble ack-ack responded because most everything had moved north. The fuel dump exploded. Huge flames billowed up. Then the pilot sprayed the beach with his guns. The bullets ripped through where we had been. So close, but we were safe. It was scary.

Dan said there was *no* way the pilot could get back, a suicide mission. Our picnic was dampened but I had a chance to walk along the beach with Dan. The ocean was lovely, now brightly lit. It crashed onto the rocks making golden spray.

But this was good-bye to all of them, Dan, ER, Dunk, Daniel Boone and Jess, guys we had met when we first hit Leyte and who became our special friends. I'd love for you to meet all of them, so fearless, humble and yet so full of life.

Hellos and good-byes are so common here. You try to get used to them, but it is hard. These guys really adopted all five of us and their leaving hit us all hard. We pray for their safety!!

Work is very hard and challenging but I am proud of this hospital. There is a real *esprit de corps* here. We've become a real unit and work well together and respect each other. That is good.

Happy Easter to you both! I'm waiting to get home, but it will be a while! I've been overseas seven months and am I yellow!!! …

Love, Sally B.

March 15, 1945

Dear Mom and Dad,

Another week has flown by. I'm so very busy on Ward #25. Bruno has made a garden on each side of our path to the ward. We've planted vegetables and marigolds, zinnias and delphinium! What fun. I'm so lucky Captain McKay let Bruno and Bannister transfer to me from Ward #16 to Ward #25. It has made all the difference to all of us.

Sunday night I went with BC, June and Tommy (*Lucia Tomkins*) to sing in a chapel near the airstrip. We practiced after work on Sunday, "Finlandia" and "Now that Day is Over." ... The Chaplain came to get us. We went to the loveliest chapel made of bamboo and with some illuminated windows. We were the only ladies and were nervous but it was really fun to sing in this chapel choir. We hope to get a larger group for Easter. I told the padre I'd work on it. A photographer took a picture of the choir.

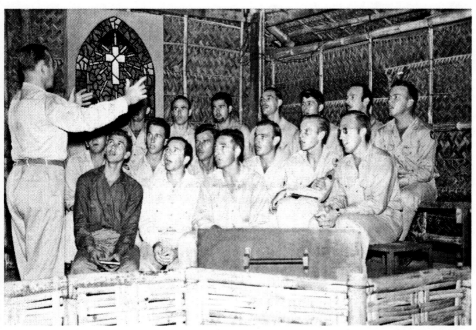

The man in the back row, on the far right, painted the stained glass windows. There were three windows in all.

Surprise, Dan showed up two nights ago. I was so surprised and happy. I don't know how he works these trips, but I'm glad he does. We had another wonderful evening talking.

By the way, I just got a lovely package from Grampus — Shraft's candies, a detective story and a flashlight. It was sent to an ancient APO so it was a long time coming! Everything was delicious. We all feasted and enjoyed.

Requests please:

Bras, underpants, face powder, nail polish and remover, bobby pins, any canned milk or meat, nail scissors, stationery and airmail stamps — Thank you.

Got to write a bunch of letters tonight ...

Love, Sally B.

P.S.

I've been reading a wonderful book, "The Cloister and the Hearth." It's an enchanting love story but also describes a vivid picture of medieval Holland, the home life, customs, methods of painting, apprenticeship and government. Even though it is only a novel, I can learn so much history this painless way! S.

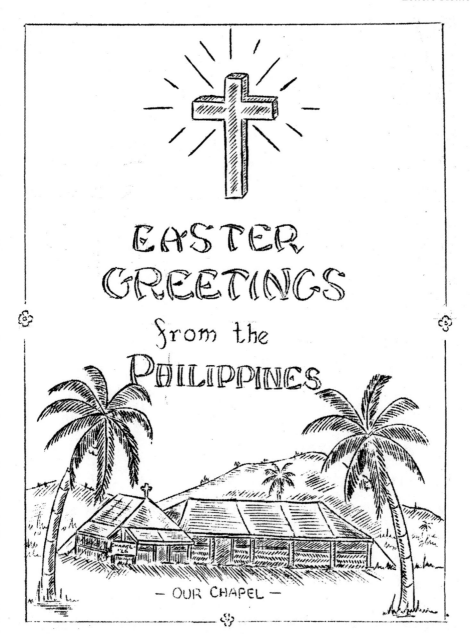

EASTER GREETINGS from the PHILIPPINES

— OUR CHAPEL —

The 43rd Bombardment Group Choir sang for Easter Services on Sunday, March 11, 1945 in the chapel pictured on page 129. BC, Junie, Tommy Tompkins and I were the guest quartet from the 126th General Hospital that evening. We stood and sang where the men are sitting here. The Chaplain who conducted the services was John H. Huston.

March 21, 1945

Dear Mom and Dad,

… A very busy week. Saturday night was the formal opening of the Officers' Club here at the hospital. We all had a wonderful time at the dance. Believe it or not, I danced so much to the nickelodeon that my feet were sore, even in my high Army shoes!! A far cry from the tent, the logs and boxes!

Every other night after work June and Betty and I have been out playing in our convalescent area, badminton, baseball and basketball. It's a good feeling to be out doing sports and to stretch the body and to get tired. This hospital is getting so civilized!!

The other night I went out with an Aussie officer. It was different. I got a real lesson on Australian geography — and a long dissertation on the future of his country, its medical potentials and business futures, and his own ideas of America! I was shocked. He said he pitied America and its Negro problem.

It seemed frightening somehow to hear him say that. I know how angry I felt when I hit the attitude of discrimination that was so blatant when I worked on the Officers' Ward in New Guinea. And I realize I almost never see black faces here, at least not in the hospital.

I feel so strongly that prejudice is WRONG. I wish I could do something. Remember how moved I was in school when I read Richard Wright's "Black Boy" and "12 Million Black Voices," where he sums up the attitude of Negroes by asking not "Can I Do It?" but "Will They Let Me Do It?" What a terrible situation for a man overseas fighting for his country to feel that he's doing his part, but wonders whether he will face the same discriminatory pre-war attitudes when he gets home.

I was deeply troubled by my discussion and embarrassed. I know it's wrong to discriminate. It's awful to feel another country's pity!

The ward is hectic with so many different doctors on so many different services but it is a real challenge and I do love it. I'm still working overtime each day. Why I went out to play two hours of hard sports — who knows?? After doing my laundry, I was ready to hit the sack and I did.

P.S. my APO is changed! APO 72 has been split. Now I'm APO 1004!!!

Love, Sally B.

March 29, 1945

Hi Folks,

… Got my <u>first</u> afternoon off. Hooray!! The hospital arranged for us nurses, Betty, BC, Mickey, Shirl and me, and others, to go to the beach to swim in the wide Pacific with its breakers! I'm such a novice!! I don't understand the ocean, being a mountain lake person myself. I got gently tossed and scraped and bruised, but it was lots of fun, the most I've had since Dan and his friends left. We were able to swim from 2 to 5 p.m. We had air mattresses and we played tag and leapfrog. What a wonderful treat!!

The week has flown by. I'm now teaching classes of Filipino girls on my floor. They are eager to help and I'm giving classes in basic care, beds, changing water, cleaning stands, and even enemas. Their extra hands will be so very useful. We need MANY extra hands!!

A couple of nights ago, Dick M., a Naval officer we all knew well on the *Holbrook* came calling again. (He's the one who knows Aunty Ruth and Uncle Bob.) He took me to his ship for supper. We had steaks, ice cream and fruit salad. There was a tablecloth on the table, silverware and glasses. Just three weeks ago we stopped eating out of our mess kits!! It was a real treat to eat like a lady again. The Navy eats well and lives well!!

Victory!! Two days ago, Bruno pulled the first radishes from our garden. We've been nursing them along for a few weeks. They are HOT!! Must say I'll not eat too many! Then the directive came from on high. "Do NOT eat any *uncooked* foods from the ground or any foods not covered by skins!" (The *contaminated soil posed a health risk.*) No salad greens for us!! No radishes!! What a bummer!!

The flowers are coming along. Our little ward should be pretty soon!!

BC and I have both heard from Dan and ER. They are so courageous! What a terrible thing to have to face this new onslaught for the fifth time. We all pray for all of them ... (*They were on their way to Okinawa. The invasion began on April 1, 1945*)

Love Sally B.

March 29, 1945

Dear Mom and Dad,

… Got a long letter from brother John yesterday and I wrote a long one back because he had written me about the value and fallacies of the world in which we live. I do not agree entirely with him in that our generation's values are all up for redefinition. I feel there are basic values and standards set up by society that never need redefining, but maybe some do.

I argued for pages about that and then began my theories on a better post-war world. I stressed that I feel our educational system today is inadequate. I feel that theoretical education should begin long before college is reached. Youth needs to learn to think, and think clearly. They need to be given tools to work with. They need to have tools of living so that they can marry long before the present educational system allows.

Mom and Dad, how's this for being steamed up on ideas? So much to think about!

Love, Me

April through June
Adventure to Carigara

April 5th, 1945

Dear Mom and Dad,

… A lot of things have been happening this past week. Carl R. took June and me exploring in his jeep. Carl is in the Signal Corps and comes from Denver. He is like a brother to me and my pals. He plays the guitar, sings, is jolly, kind, thoughtful, and always eager to take us where we want to go in his jeep. He let us both drive it. I wore his helmet, which was so big it sat on my head like a basket, so I was inconspicuous!!

He took us also to see how he makes his maps. He is a cartographer. We saw how they print maps, reduce them, add color and all the delicate work that goes into producing a map from a series of airplane photos. Remember when I first was in nursing school, I was asked to come to Washington to serve in the US Coast and Geodetic Survey to help with maps because I'd had that cartography course at Smith reading aerial maps? Seems so long ago. I'm glad I stayed in nursing school!

This week was one of HUGE surprises. John Reed came for a visit. (*A neighbor from the town I grew up in, Bristol Connecticut.*) I haven't seen Johnny for ten years, I'll bet! He's a lieutenant on an LST, still big, jolly, full of fun and news of Bristol. He told me about seeing Bill Duquette (*a neighbor and friend of my brother's in Bristol*) who is here and a T/Sgt. It's been years since I've seen these old neighborhood friends.

But yesterday was the special day because it was a real adventure. Carl said the road over the mountain to Carigara on the north coast was safe to drive. So, he wanted to take me. It was my second afternoon off since January.

The day was crystal clear. We rode through rice paddies. On our left were high green mountain peaks holding shelves of gray blue clouds. Filipino men and women in their huge sun hats were cutting rice in their fields. Farmers were riding in their carts behind their slow plodding carabao along the side of the road. There were many flowers, red, yellow, blue and white growing in clusters under the graceful palms.

We drove through some little towns. Guess it was siesta time because men seemed to be asleep on their store counters. Women were talking to some GIs. Little kids jumped and screamed "Vic-to-ry" as we passed. We came upon an old cathedral. It was not in good repair. A man and his patient carabao stood outside. We stopped to take his picture.

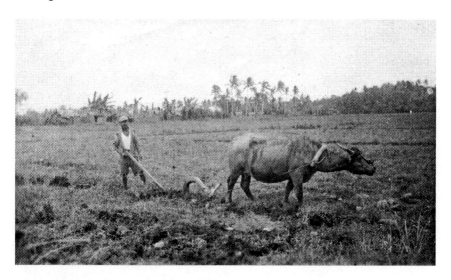

Tilling the land with a wooden plow.

The landscape changed from the broad flat valley to a more mountainous New England-like terrain. There were small plots of harrowed land being tilled by a man holding a crude wooden plow, pulled by his carabao. We think this is for sugar cane. We took a picture of this old man plowing his field.

Army vehicles grew scarcer, GIs too. The road grew narrow and bumpy as it followed a swift-moving stream. When we passed people some called, "Americans, Victory!" Some children were flying kites.

Over the mountain on the other side, Carigara appeared ahead of us. It was so quaint with its narrow, twisting streets. There were carts full of coconuts and hemp. Carts moved to the side of the road as we went by. Stores lined the roads, displaying dried fish, hats, wooden clogs, rice bread and bananas. As we wound through the streets, there, before us was the ocean, a lovely big bay.

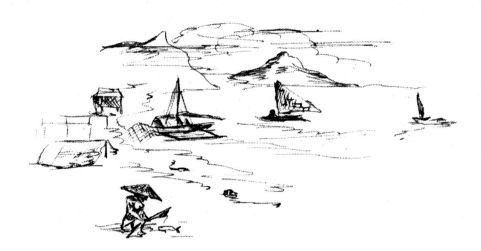

View of Carigara Harbor

It was full of large and small outriggers with bright sails. Many people were busy with their nets. Pigs and dogs roamed at will. Rice lay on mats made of mesh, drying. We got out to walk along the shore behind the drying hemp nets. Golden-brown people were tending to their chores as they had for centuries.

"Hello," we heard and turned to see a smiling woman in a bright blue dress waving to us. "Do you want to buy a grass skirt?" We wandered toward her as she held up a gaudy red and green hemp job.

"How much?"

"Ten peso!" We didn't want it.

"But you want some necklace?"

She held up a handful of exquisite shell chains. They were white and delicate and smelled of fish.

"They are lovely," I exclaimed.

"To you, you take six chains for five pesos!" So I thanked her and paid for them.

"What's your name, nurse?"

"Sally," I said. Gales of laughter from three generations of onlookers.

"I am Mrs. Alfredo Farrantes!" We all smiled.

"You will come again?" she asked.

"No, I think we won't."

"Well, you come to see me, if you do." It had been a friendly exchange.

We saw men making hemp ropes that were then wound onto a spool by a man turning a wheel. Another man was sorting fibers. Children and women peered shyly at us. Not too many visitors had come here as yet.

We saw a pair of carved sandals. "Try them, Sal," Carl suggested. So, I held them up to my foot. "Oh, Carl, they are too small!" A little girl in a white embroidered dress looked on hoping for a sale, then — "Too small. JESUS CHRIST, what a foot!"

This from this little girl. We both laughed, it was so unexpected. I took my boot off and tried on the sandal. Again, "Jesus Christ, what a foot!" Obviously, no sale, but she gave us two bananas and began to sing, "Pistol Packing Mama!" She'd met Americans before!

Slowly we drove through the busy town to the outskirts where there was a storybook old Spanish church covered with moss and shaded by huge, gnarled oak-like trees. We went inside. Dim light filtered through the cracked and boarded up windows but we could see the old carvings and a painted altar. An old wall outside, attached to the church, enclosed the monks' and nuns' garden. It was still intact but starting to crumble.

We drove along the beach, racing the incoming tide and setting sun. Women waved and went back to sorting their rice. It is flipped over and over again onto a mat. The chaff flows out like golden smoke around their legs. The little children in their tops and no bottoms jumped up to see us. We drove over narrow bridges past a swamp where some carabao lay half in and half out of the mud chewing their cuds. One little fellow scampered away, tail in the air, then turned to view us with a big question in his eyes!

The sky was growing red and the world around us pink, so we turned around to head back. It was a beautiful sight, the blue-green sea with its lacy white edges pushing onto the land then pulling out to try again. The beach we drove on was blue-black. White shells and coconuts broke its monotony. It was so strange. We were so close to the war, yet seemed so removed, another age, another land, until I saw to my right a sign, "Mrs. Gorodin's Machineless Waves!" Will wonders never cease?

We sped back to town, over the rickety little bridge and out of town where the pigs and chickens and the families lived together with the patient carabao, away from the sunset, east, to the shore area where we were all encamped.

The mountains grew darker. The sea sounds faded. Our adventure was done, except that the memories of this first Leyte adventure away from our eastern shore would last me a lifetime.

It was 50 miles to Carl's place where we had supper. We drove up his hill and saw the main harbor full of ships so different from those fishing outriggers we had just seen. Cars and trucks sped along on the road below us. We looked down at the trees below which so recently had had their tops blown off by mortars.

I thanked Carl for being such a good friend. He is like a brother to me. A very thoughtful, kind man, considerate and good. I'm lucky to have such a friend.

To top the day, we saw the movie, "A Song to Remember," about Chopin's life. Beautiful music. What an end to my first Leyte adventure! …

> Love, Sally B.

April 14, 1945

Dear Mom and Dad,

… What a shock to the world, Roosevelt's death! He had become a symbol of freedom and to all of us, THE LEADER. I know our country will go on, but who is this Harry Truman? I wonder what he has done, what he believes. Will he be a strong leader in our post-war world? Will he be able to cope with the Russians? With all Roosevelt's imperfections, he did represent our free world. The world's nations trusted him. He symbolized USA. However, I believe he will go down in history with Washington and Lincoln as one of our great leaders who has piloted us through many of our most turbulent years. He seemed far ahead of his times in thoughts and ideas. His ideas were theoretically for the common man. He's left behind him many ideas and special programs for the common man, and a great pride in our country. So goes a great humanitarian!! And a GREAT LEADER!

Oh, well, I'm on nights again, my third night assignment. Wonder what will happen this time?!! It's a good change, but it's so hard to sleep, it's so hot.

Betty has a friend, Junior, who flies a Piper Cub[14] called "Sad Sack." Anyway, Junior took Betty and me up sightseeing. Oh, I love to fly!! We flew over our whole area, saw the mortar and shell scars, trenches and topless trees. He flew low up the valley with its rice paddies, its furrowed fields, palm trees and the spine of the green and purple mountains. It's hard to believe there were Japs here not long ago and that there are still some cut off in the mountains. The scars from the fighting are still so clear in the holes in the green fields!

Junior went low over some carabao trying to make them move, but they chewed placidly on and never batted an eye. Maybe they are deaf. We're told they are strange. They supposedly hate white people and are docile as lambs with their owners. I have no proof of this theory!!

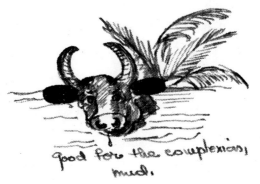

good for the complexion, mud.

Good for the complexion — mud! A caribao.

We're able to go swimming more often now. The hospital arranges transportation to take us in the afternoon. I've turned very brown. It covers the saffron yellow from the atabrine.

[14] A small one-engine plane.

We have a wonderful hospital. How lucky we are. The nurses, WACs and ARC[15] staff are so compatible, and all the medical staff and enlisted men are a wonderful team!!

Well, eight months on April 21st!!

Still no word from Dan and the friends who went to Okinawa. It's scary!!

Love, Sally B.

Amoeba

April 18, 1945

Dear Mom and Dad,

… It's a beautiful day today, warm and rather like those summer days at home when the family would pack up a picnic basket, pile into the car, and drive out to the country to enjoy! I can still smell the hay this time of year. I remember it looks like water, rippling in the wind, all yellow, red and gold mixed in the green, hay that's full of plantain, devil's paint brush, buttercups and daisies. Definitely not a good hay, but it sure is beautiful! Funny how certain days recall to mind other associations.

Today I have great plans for letter writing, reading, and even making some sketches because now I will have time to do many things. You know I really enjoyed my week on nights. My third night assignment lasted only seven days. The first time we shipped

---

[15] American Red Cross

out of Devens, the second to the Philippines and this time I'm in the hospital with amoebic dysentery.

It was a strange week on nights; seven to seven is a long haul. We had so many chores to do, transfer all orders, sort and file all lab slips, give all medications. Between 3 and 4 a.m., there was a terrible need to sleep so the ward men would go to the mess hall and bring back old boiled coffee. I'll never forget that coffee, but it cured sleepiness.

At 7 a.m. I have morning report, then breakfast, a shower and bed in our night nurses quarters before it got too hot to sleep.

Did I tell you about breakfasts? We grab our trays with dividers onto which we serve ourselves pancakes or dry cereal with canned milk. The pancakes are at least an inch thick and doughy and the syrup is so sweet. Butter is canned. We've never found out how or why it seems to always taste rancid. But the coffee was great!! We all take our atabrine and salt pills then go off for the day's work after scraping our trays into a big can and dipping them into another can of hot garbagey water. This always seems gross to me for the hot water is gray with food floating on the top. So much for breakfast.

After breakfast I go to my tent, peel off all my clothes, usually wet with sweat, and take my Army issue, seersucker wraparound uniform which I use for a bathrobe, and head down the wooden path to the showers.

I keep my old uniform, now a bathrobe, hanging on the T-bar at the foot of my bed. One morning last week when I discarded my nightclothes, I put on the wraparound and felt something BIG moving on my leg! I pulled the front open. There was an enormous 6" hairy spider half on my leg and half on the robe. I'm afraid I screamed! I yanked the robe off, brushed that THING off me and ran emotionally down that path to the shower with nothing on at all!

The sweet little Filipino girl who does our laundry was on her way to our tent and saw me behaving hysterically. She saw the spider and stepped on it!! She was barefoot! Then, bless her heart, she followed me to the shower with my robe and a towel. I was really ashamed of myself but it was rather awful and funny I guess for anyone who may have seen me racing stark naked through the nurses' area as if the demons or Japanese had been after me!! So much for that.

Sleeping days in the Nipa-roofed sleeping quarters is no fun. I rush through breakfast, my shower and hurry to bed. Shaded as it is by the big jungle trees and roofed with thatch, it is still hot. By noon we are often in 100-degree humid heat. We lie on the sheets with no covers and soak the bed. By noon or 1 p.m. I wake up unable to sleep anymore.

Sometimes in these afternoons, we who are on nights get to go swimming on the beach several miles south at the Officers' Club. We are taken by an arranged vehicle from the hospital.

The club is in a beautiful spot with palms waving at the edge of the wide, sandy beach. The club is a simple structure at the edge of the beach and under the trees. (*All I remember about those swims is how warm and how gentle is the Pacific, most of the time.*) I love the sea here.

The beach shelves very slowly out for a long way so the wave action is gentle. It is refreshing and treasured for it is such an occasional treat.

On nights last week, I began to have terrible abdominal cramps. "Oh, boy," I thought, "I wonder what is the trouble this time? You went off night's last time, you can't do it again!"

The cramps were awful. Sleeping was a problem for I had developed the "runs" too. So, I told my supervisor how I felt. "You are always sick on nights!! You can't get sick now," I was told, "we have so many sick to care for and we're so short of staff." We had over 2800 instead of 1500!! So — I went back on duty at 7 p.m. I remember that night. I was sitting at my desk doing deskwork holding a hot water bottle on my stomach. It was not a bit professional. Then I kept running over to the nurses' latrine where I had extreme diarrhea and weakness, but I came back hoping it would all go away.

I'm still not sure why Dr. Lewis,[16] who was doing detached service from the Navy on my floor, arrived at 5:30 a.m. to ask me about my floor (I always suspected Sgt. Bruno!). But he also asked about me, how long I'd had symptoms, what they were and then he said I was to give him a stool sample that he would take to the lab. "NOW!!." He drew blood saying I was so white, he was worried.

---

[16] Commanders Lewis and Besseson were both Navy doctors serving with the 126th until the Navy hospital on Samar was done. Both were excellent physicians and great friends. They both took wonderful care of all my women and me.

So, easily, I obliged with the sample, went to breakfast, the showers, and finally to bed in the sleeping quarters. I was drifting off when we were all startled to see Dr. Lewis in our sleeping quarters.

We looked up amazed. He came straight to me, picked me up in my sheet and told me I was going to the hospital — that I was very sick with acute, severe amoebic dysentery. He carried me over in his arms. I was admitted here on my own Ward, #25.

And so I begin to be a hospital patient myself.

Love, Sally B.

I remember —

My stay lasted much too long. I didn't get out for four weeks — from April 16-May 13! I was not alone. Amoebic dysentery was all too common throughout the southwest Pacific area and among our hospital staff.

Amoebic dysentery is caused by a one-celled animal, the amoeba, which lives in the human bowel and bores into the lining making ulcers. Unclean hands, contaminated soil or water, uncooked foods, open latrines and flies are the common means of contamination.

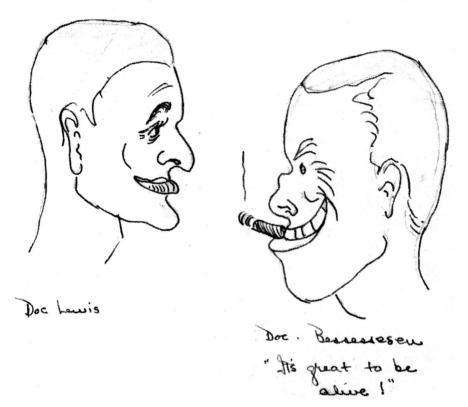

Doc Lewis

Doc. Bersessesew
"It's great to be alive!"

Symptoms varied from mild diarrhea to abdominal pain, cramps and bloody diarrhea. Patients were treated with emetine, a drug given twice daily intra-muscularly, for ten days. Because the therapeutic dose was so close to the toxic dose, we were all kept in bed. There were side effects for some of us — nausea, extreme muscular weakness and rapid heartbeat, but these side effects passed.

Two other drugs, carbarsone and diodoquin, followed after the live amoeba were killed by emetine. Today, antibiotics simplify and shorten this second-stage treatment following emetine. I have no idea when or how so many others and I contracted this misery, but it was a real problem which affected many of our hospital staff.

April 19, 1945

Dear Folks,

… Your birthday box came yesterday, before the big day. Thanks for the peanuts, bath powder, cold cream and toothpaste all beautifully wrapped. What a surprise. Thank you so very much.

It's strange to be a bed patient on my own floor, but everyone is so nice and helpful. Johnny Reed came again bearing a crate of orange juice, pineapple juice and some canned chicken. Nothing like the Navy sharing with the Army. He's been so kind. I'm glad his Mom and you are such good friends. It has helped me here, anyway.

At least I'm glad the awful cramping is less, but the trots are a nuisance. I'll have to have 10 days of intra-muscular treatment to kill the live forms of the amoeba. Then days of heavy metals to kill the eggs. Oh, well! This will be my time to rest and read.

Love, Sally B.

April 20, 1945

Dear Mom and Dad,

… I'm twenty-six today. Here I am in bed!! But what a day I had. I've had callers all day, the man in admissions office came, and Johnny Reed came again bearing more juices. He's so kind. This morning, Mercedes, my tent Filipino girl, the heroine who squashed the tarantula, came with a huge bouquet of red, pink, yellow, white flowers. Carl came, after sending a singing telegram. Dr. Besseson and Dr. Lewis of course are here on detached service, so they had to bring a laugh or two.

Dr. Lewis is married to a Smith girl, Class of 1939. She lived at Gardner and 17 Henshaw. Small world! I've been with him to 7th Fleet HQ to parties. He and his buddy, Dr. "Bess" Besseson, also Navy, have been so supportive on Ward #25. They are taking very good care of me.

We've had NO word from Dan, ER or any of those wonderful guys who left here mid-March. We know now that the invasion of Okinawa began on April 1. We are all anxious about them.

We know many of our men are still mopping up these Philippine Islands. Our hospital is bulging. We've had almost 3,000 census. We were geared for 1,500.

Before I was admitted last week, I met a captain from the US Coast and Geodetic Survey. He had come straight from the States. How we laughed, he was so pink and white. We remembered how the nurses laughed at us in Hollandia when we first landed. He also laughed now at how yellow we are!! Good fun.

Love, Me

April 22, 1945

Dear Folks,

… There is much to tell you tonight. I have become a complete bed patient because of the drug emetine. I was grounded when April 20th rolled around.

It was a wonderful birthday for me, one of the most wonderful and humbling in all my 26 years. Betty came on her way to work with a bottle of shampoo, Shirl with an honest-to-goodness orange, toothpaste, a can of fruit juice and a big hug. That began it all with a bang.

Bruno's and my flowers, which we had planted weeks ago, were in full bloom. The two Navy doctors on my floor left a lovely printed scarf on my bed — "To a marvelous girl, from the Navy!" They are so kind and such good doctors.

After breakfast I got all my medicine which included my morning shot of emetine in my fanny. I'm so full of shots! Two weeks of penicillin every four hours and now two intra-muscular shots of emetine each day for ten days. I'm a real speckled hen. It's not easy finding a spot to inject, so I just turn over and say, "Go ahead. You're bound to use one of the original holes, so what the dickens!" Every day is one day less and nearer to the end of the emetine which makes me sick. I've lost weight!!

All through the day the kids came in and out. The kids came in with the PX. I had to have an extra board put under my bed to hold everyone's generosity. I've decided I need a branch office! Johnny Reed came yet again bearing all kinds of canned foods and juices, full of laughs and good nature.

The climax came when Shirl, June, BC, Betty, Mickey and dates arrived bearing the biggest cake I've ever seen! It was 18 inches by 18 inches and three layers high — all decorated with beige frosting, pink roses, green leaves, and "Happy Birthday, Sally" written on top. An iced cake!! I could hardly keep from crying.

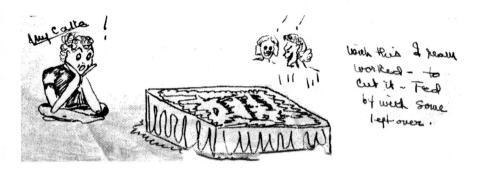

Well Johnny Reed cut it up and served everyone on the ward and their visitors. It was such a happy occasion only dampened by the fact that none of us has word from Okinawa from Dan and his friends. We are so afraid of what that means …

Yesterday I found out! Dan did get it. He was shot through the shoulder and has a fractured left arm, a bayonet wound in his right arm and bullet wounds in his right hand. He was shot through his chest and stomach, but is alive and he'll be sent home.

First, his friend Lt. Landmesser wrote me (a letter I got on April 20th) that on April 5, "Dan picked you a big bouquet of flowers. He'll write himself soon." (*"Flowers" was a code Dan and I had set up so that I would know when there had been an injury.*)

Then a letter from Dan came to me stating how it happened.

He states, "I walked into a cave after those jokers, but a clip hit before I could say 'hello.' Didn't like that, so I went in after him. Got some more clips, my arm broke so I dropped my gun. Had a brawl and kept the bayonet from getting me. Then up comes Lt. Landmesser (*the one who wrote me about Dan*) and lets go with his 45. Thought it was about time to get the hell out. So we ran and ran, yelled like hell for the aid man because I was about to fall on my head. Got operated on in an hour! So, Sal, I got my Purple Heart and I'm going home, not the way I wanted but I'm the luckiest guy alive. They took my picture because I'm the first guy to have so many bullets and still be alive. See, my 'lucky star' again! Gave you straight stuff because I promised. It will take me a while to heal …" He said he had his picture taken because never had a soldier with so much lead in him lived to tell the tale!

The other gals have had letters from some of the others up there. ER and Dunk have made it so far. What a terrible war when all these wonderful guys have to go through such HELL! (*All returned home but Jesse.*)

As for me, this business is not the breeze I thought it would be. Dr. Heath offered to evacuate me because of my boils but I refused. I'm needed here so much. We have such a heavy patient load and here I am cooling my heels in bed when everyone else is working so hard. I just feel this hospital is where I belong. This is my little war, but it's a h— of a way to fight it. I hope I'll be up soon.

Must be forsythia and daffy time at home with tulips to follow. I can remember so well helping Dad uncover the bulbs. Soon the trees will burst out and the air will be full of spring and birds. It's getting to be spring here too, then summer. We are all getting used to the heat …

Love, Sally B.

April 25th, 1945

Dear Mom and Dad,

… Thanks so very much for the food package and the books besides my lovely birthday box. I've told you the emetine makes me sick but my friend, Lt. R. Rassmusson, a WAC on the floor with me, Dr. Lewis, Shirl and I sat around and had some of your soup with noodles, turkey and fruit. What a treat. I did eat. It was fun. Still a bed patient.

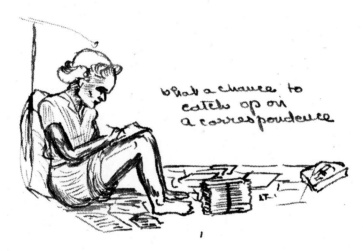

what a chance to catch up on a correspondence

Miss McKay asked again when I'm to get out. Who knows? I've got to have three negative specimens before I can move! It's a real experience to be a bed patient. All nurses should try it once. Many lessons to be remembered …

… You know that lying here in my sack, I get a wonderful bird's-eye view of the world outside. This morning two of the little evacueé kids were out playing, the Russian boy about six, the American about four. The littler shaver had on a long pair of corduroy overalls, quite big. When he ran along beside his bigger hero, he looked rather like a teddy bear.

Well, the six-year-old stepped over a ditch and reached for a butterfly. The little one charged up behind him, stopped at the ditch, then tried to jump. His pants were too long, the ditch too big and the child too small — all added up to a magnificent four-point landing. He got up, looked around for some adult to cuddle him. No one, so he charged after his hero laughing and screaming.

The little Russian boy is the one who threw me for a loop the night of my birthday. After all the visitors had left and most of the cake had been shared with all the other patients, I went down to #15 bed. The net was down on the bed. I thought McCloskey must be having malaria.[17]

"Hey, gal, want some cake?" One eye peered out from under the sheet. McCloskey had shrunk in size!! Suddenly, a small body appeared. It was the young boy! What a surprise! It's fun to see kids around!

Love, Me

April 26, 1945

Dear Mom and Dad,

… Time in bed gives me all kinds of flights of imagination. As I was lying quietly looking up at the superstructure of the tent above me, I began to observe a Gecko catching bugs on the main support. He was zooming from one end of the ridgepole to the other snapping

---

[17] All malaria patients were screened at night to protect them from mosquitoes and us from being bitten by infected mosquitoes.

away, filling his stomach. Along came a butterfly, teasing, just out of reach and stayed just out of reach until it flew away.

Soon, amazingly, there was a general assembly, lizards of all colors chasing up and down the tent pole like those electric charge boxes on tracks in department stores. That continued. Then came some call to attention.

All the cavorting ceased. The ranks lined up for some speech on laxity in the younger generation. I was hit in the face by a tear from one of the culprits (I hope it was a tear). The elder continued. Only the back row moved, catching mosquitoes.

After it was all over, off they went making their queer but distinctive "gecko" noise. Only the old one stayed put over my bed. I'm sure he shook his head at the youngsters. He was still there this morning.

But this morning a new one came right up the pole next to my bed post, looked around, winked, stuck out his tongue, flipped his tail, and with the old one, both were gone. I was so surprised I didn't even jump. Sat there like the bed patient I am and stared!

Just finished reading "Precious Bane" by Webb. It's a different and lovely story. The descriptions of hay and haying rang a bell in my heart. It described walking through the hay field, the grass being long and soft. And I remembered how our shoes used to get filled with pollen. How we'd look back to see the wake we'd made which didn't all close behind us and how mad the farmer would be because we'd knocked down his crop! It's a lovely story about a terrible handicap and real love and appreciation!

Just a note to close. I bought two pairs of Australian-made female slacks. I was pleased to know I'd have extras. Tried them on. I can't win. The legs are miles too long; the crotch comes to my knees. I'm sure I'll trip, as one leg catches into the other leg if I bend my knees. I do need a tailor! Until then, I'll have to continue to wear my forbidden men's pants until I am chastised for being out of uniform! Oh, my!

Love, Sally B.

April 26, 1945

Dear Aunt Helen,

… When I wrote you from Hollandia, I said I was busy. We were, but I didn't know what busy meant then. We are all working so very hard now. We need more nurses and here I am a bed patient. I know my being here puts a big extra load on all the rest. We have quite a few nurses sick here now. We are all exhausted.

Our hospital is beautiful! When we came it was a drained swamp with carabao popping out of mud wallows. That was the rainy season. What a transformation! Now we have tarred roads, a huge hospital, some tent wards (medical), some prefabs (surgical). We have a convalescent area made from the old swamp, which now is beautiful. We also have a baseball diamond, badminton courts, a bowling alley, and basketball courts. The buildings are brightly painted. What a joy a week spent here must be for those guys who have been so sick and who've come here to get better …

Love, Sally

April 30, 1945

Dear Mom,

Your natal day comes up on the 18th of May. I had to write to wish you a wonderful Happy Day. Please take some money out of my account and buy something you really want. Just know I admire you and Dad. You are both so gutsy and I'm lucky to have you for a Mom!!

Surprise. Bill Duquette popped in on me two nights ago. It's been years, twelve, I guess, since I saw Bill and played softball in the vacant lot with the neighborhood gang! Johnny Reed told him I was here. It is so nice to have old neighbors take the time and trouble to look in to say "hello." How small a world!!

Doc Lewis is coming around. He says to say "hello" and tell you I'm a good patient! He's taking very good care of me.

Oh, and Mom, thanks to both of you for the package that came yesterday. Heaven Scent bath powder and the book "Storm." I shall dazzle everyone with the smell.

With much love, Sally

May 3, 1945

Dear Folks,

We are all relieved that most of the guys in Okinawa are all right. Dan is in a cast on his way to Saipan. A funny letter arrived from him. What a great guy and a wonderful sport. He's on his way home!

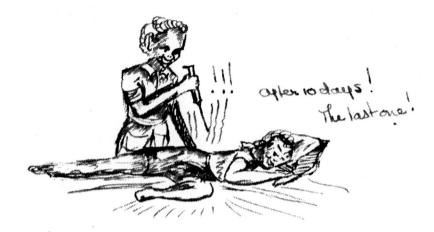

I'm still here! I'm still longing to get out. Three nights ago a guy who works in surgery gave me a wonderful gift. I was allowed out of bed, so I went to the movies, but I felt as though I was walking on golf balls. On my way home, this med tech gave me a *cot mattress* for my canvas cot. Remember when, at the start, the hospital was so flooded with patients that we nurses gave our real beds up to the hospital? The mattress was a BIG event like the pail was in Hollandia!! I'm so fortunate!!

When I got back to the ward, all I wanted was to put on my PJs and hit the sack. I stood outside to brush my teeth. Something was stuck in my pajama leg. A centipede! I shook my leg hard, uttered a canned squeal and shook again. I heard it land! Then I heard another squeal. Quigley had one on her neck. If you think we crawled into bed without looking under everything, you're wrong! This ward has turned into a lizards' and centipedes' paradise!!! Oh, I do so want to get out!

Last night a Navy friend of Dr. Lewis' brought me a pail of celery, real celery, heads, hearts and all. Went around offering some to everyone. I felt like St. Nicholas. It was so good, crisp, ice cold, and such a treat. People are so very kind and nice!

Love, Me

May 6, 1945

Dear Mom and Dad,

I asked again when I was to get out, and Dr. Lewis said, "Oh, you'll be out in time for the Yale-Harvard Game!" Frustration!

Hooray! Last night I got a pass. I went to a steak roast on the beach with Dr. Lewis, Dr. Bess, Shirl, BC and Lt. Brain, cooked steaks and onions and roasted potatoes done in the coals, the way we did at home across the street. It was SO good, thanks to the Navy. But I was so glad to get back to bed.

Yesterday, I had an invitation from a Captain James Smith, USN to join him for a meal on his ship, the *Admiral Hershey*! He told my chief nurse he knew you two. WHO is he? Am I supposed to know him? I can't get out of bed for that long anyway.

Just got word about Germany. IT'S OVER AT LAST!! Brother John can come home and all our other friends over there. *How absolutely wonderful it's over.* Thank God!! Maybe now they can send some more men and machines over here. We sure could use some help to end this bloody, gruesome war, so our guys can go home and begin to live their lives again! May it be soon!! How wonderful to have PEACE in Europe!!

Still reading all I can get my hands on! Just finished reading "The Pacific World" telling a lot about geology, botany, and anthropology on the islands. It was abbreviated but good. Need more information. Am reading Somerset Maughan's "Theatre." Characterizations are wonderful but not too appealing. Gives a peculiar impression about the way so many we know live, a good way, but not very real!

What a surprise, I will get out this week!! But I am so weak. I trust it is only sitting around doing nothing for so long.

Love, Sally B.

May 10, 1945

Dear Mom and Dad,

On Saturday I will be discharged! Before I am, I was told to get my teeth checked. It has been a year, so I had them cleaned. No cavities, but I have two impacted lower wisdom teeth. Action — the dentist took out my lower left using a riveting machine, pound, pound, swear, pound, pound, twist — 'Hooray, half out!' Pound a few times more and the other half came out. It was over after a few stitches. I tried to smile. Only half of my face worked. Ridiculous! Came back to Ward #25, played a bit of bridge, took some codeine, and went to sleep on an ice bag.

Was awakened by a chorus from "Oklahoma!!" The USO show was with us. Two of the women in the cast are in bed on our floor. Shirley Jones, the star, is in the bed next to me. She's so warm and sweet!

In the late morning, some of the cast came to Ward #25 to sing a few numbers. They sat all over the beds and sang. The Persian Peddler sat on my bed, going through his silly routine. He was a bit obnoxious, but the music is SO catchy!!

Yesterday I found out why I was so weak! I was terribly anemic so I got a pint of some nice person's blood and I feel wonderful!! I got up afterwards and went to a basketball game, and then went to see the movie "National Velvet" with the gang.

Just finished reading "Valley of Decision" by Marcia Davenport. It was fun and a real education about the early industrial growth in America, the money involved, the unions that sprang up, the need for social welfare work. It is a multi-generational saga, the loves, hates, pride, hopes and fears in two families, one the industrialist and the other the worker. Both are tied together by one Irish Catholic maid, Mary Rafferty who lives through many generations. I've never read a book that describes the early American industrial scene so completely.

It is getting hotter, but my zinnias are beautiful! Who would have dreamed they'd do so well out here?! They are all colors, rose, yellow, lavender, red, and coral. It's very welcoming to my floor!!

Love, Sally B.

May 12, 1945

Dear Mom and Dad,

I read a wonderful book today, "Immortal Wife" by Irving Stone. It's the life of John and Jessie Fremont. There is something beautiful in the life of that man and woman, what their marriage was and what it became. There was one paragraph I shall never forget.

After 50 years of married life, John goes away to die alone and Jessie, his wife, couldn't understand this, but deep down she knew.

"She had thought of this as a failure in her marriage. Now she realized that no one can ever completely understand another human soul. What was important was not the whole and total finding, the search, the sympathy, the ever present and loving desire to understand. That, in its last analysis, was what love was, when viewed over half a century: at first it was light hearted romance, then it was physical mating, then it was ambition and work together, then it was raising a family and creating a home, then it was service in good and various causes, then it was a mature partnership in progress and accomplishment, failure and hardship. Yes, love changed subtly with the passage of the years, but lasting longest and having the deepest meaning, creating the finest hours and the finest years was the search for understanding, the full and sympathetic understanding of another being, the most elusive and at the same time, the most beautiful of all human accomplishments. This was marriage."[18]

Isn't this beautiful? ...

Love, Sally B.

---

[18] This quote is reprinted with the kind permission of Doubleday, a division of Bantam Doubleday Dell Publishing Group, Inc. from the novel "Immortal Wife", by Irving Stone, My quote came from the 1944 edition, Doubleday Doran and Co., Inc. pp. 448-449.

Trip to the *Admiral Hershey*

May 16, 1945

Dear Mom and Dad,

… The unbelievable happened. I met your friend, Captain James Smith, USN, captain of the *Admiral Hershey*, a huge Navy transport. Major McKay had to get passes from the hospital colonel and one from the base so a friend and I could leave land to go out to the ship for dinner with the captain. She really got all this permission for Shirl and me. Dressed in our very best clothes, a high-button, long-sleeved, tan shirt, tan pants, high wool socks and high laced shoes, our heads tied up in tan wool scarves, Shirl and I were ready to go to sea!!

Promptly at 4 p.m. a lieutenant (senior grade) came for us in a Navy jeep, drove us the three-plus miles to Tacloban Harbor where we were met by a seaman and a small, fast boat which took us out a long way into Tacloban Harbor to a HUGE ship.

We were anxious! How do you greet a captain in the Navy? What to say when you don't even know him? Well, we went on and on until we arrived at this behemoth of a ship. It seemed ENORMOUS! We pulled up to a platform at the bottom of a set of LONG stairs. We looked up. There were rows of young sailors at the rail looking down, like a white fringe. We looked up at the top of those stairs. There was a small, sandy-haired man with a mustache dressed in tans.

We began to climb. I was so weak still, I wondered if I'd make it. But we both did. We climbed up and up. There at the top was the captain who held out his hand and greeted us.

"Welcome aboard, Sally! Your mother and father send their love!"

All our anxiety vanished! I introduced him to Shirl. He then took us to his quarters where we were served ice-cold Cokes. We felt very relaxed with him. He was so friendly.

Next on the agenda was a tour of his ship. First, he took us to the control rooms. Whew, how complex! Then past the gun emplacements to his hospital wards. It was so sterile! Beautiful beds with mattresses, johns, surgical rooms, ORs and a dental department. What a deal! It was fascinating. He had everyone open everything up, cupboards, rooms, everything so neat, shipshape!!

We went through his shiny kitchens. Everything was spotless and everyone seemed pleased to see the captain. After our tour we ended up in the boss's quarters with a linoleum floor, green leather cushioned chairs, and a round chromium table.

Shirl and I then went into the head (john) to wash. We turned the lock on the door. We washed Leyte's dust from our faces and hands, took off our scarves, brushed and fixed our hair, did our faces and we were ready for a Navy dinner!

We tried to unlock the door. We tried and tried. Nothing either of us did could turn that lock. We began to perspire. It was a very small space, four feet by four feet I think, anyway, sound proof, water proof. No response! We used towels, muscle, anything we could find to help unlock that door. We began to laugh. How could we possibly scream or bang on the door in the captain's quarters — and we the only women on that ship? Bad business! How to open the door? Were we to die from lack of oxygen or dissolve from the heat? We began to feel uneasy. Suddenly, something gave as we tried to force the door and both of us catapulted out of the door onto our knees before the captain, soaking wet, disheveled and laughing! We all laughed. Whatever there had been of formality and reserve was long gone! Some entrance!!

We sat down at the table covered by a white tablecloth and real napkins. First we were served a grapefruit cut like a basket and filled with orange and grapefruit sections topped with a cherry. Then came fried turkey, asparagus tips, and mashed potato in the form of a rosette, ice tea with real lemon. For dessert there was apple pie a la mode. We tried to keep the conversation on subjects other than food, but this event was so special and so different from what we were used to! The Navy lives well! And we ate from silver spoons, forks and knives!! Everything was delicious!

After supper, Captain Smith took us to his ship's store where we were told to take what we needed. We filled a bag with items hard to find in our PX, then pulled out our pesos to pay for our purchases.

"Oh no, we don't take any currency but USA money!" said the sailor in charge.

Of course the captain knew this and had the seaman put all our loot on his tab!!

It had been a wonderful adventure for us both with a very friendly man, who really went out of his way to give us hard working nurses a real break. I'm glad he was and is your friend, Mom and Dad. He was wonderful to us!! He sent his regards.[19]

The answer to one question I asked Captain Smith before we left his ship that night I'll never forget.

"Do you think we can ever win this war, Captain Smith?" I asked.

"We'll win," he answered slowly. "They are smart but we'll win because we are only a little less disorganized than they are!"

We got home to the hospital about 10:30. It was one of our real adventures over here.

Love, Me

Nurse — Surgery, Ward #6

May 20, 1945

Dear Folks,

Two days ago I went back to work — at last after too long. I was not put back on #25, my Women's Ward, but on a Men's Surgical. These guys are so young! They've only been over three or four months as replacements and are mostly 18 and 19 years old with

---

[19] I did not know then that Jimmy Smith had been captain on the aircraft carrier Hornet, sunk the 27th of October 1942 in the Solomons with a great loss of life. Jimmy and Peg, his wife, would become two special friends when my husband and I lived in Vermont.

some wicked wounds. One 19 year-old has an awful chest wound. We both work up a lather when I do his dressing. He calls me "Mom." I call him "Son." But he never lets out a whimper. They are so brave! I've developed a ward nickname — "Happy" or "Skip." It's good to be on surgery again.

One more little note for you both, Mom and Dad. Last night at supper, Major Heath, ward officer on Ward #25 came up to me and asked me when I was coming back. "I'm on Ward #6 now, Sir," I said. "Damn it," he said, "that's awful. We will miss you. You did a wonderful job!"

Wasn't that nice of him to say? I was so pleased to know I'd been appreciated there, new head nurse that I was!

It is so hot now, thunderstorms and rain. We all just pour sweat — it is very unladylike.

Oh, Mom and Dad, how sad about Hender Dye.[20]

(*He was killed April 4, 1945, in Okinawa the day before Dan was hurt.*) Hender was so sweet those nights when I took care of him in Hollandia — and so young — only 18. I do wish there would be many reinforcements put over so all this carnage would stop!!

Dan says his body cast is a pain! Soon he'll be in an airplane splint for his left arm that I gather is taking a long time to knit. He's quite blue, is really scared he will lose his arm. At least on Saipan he's part way home. His spirit is there, but dampened.

---

[20] The young soldier from Brattleboro, Vermont.

One last note, I just finished a fascinating book called "Indigo." It gives a vivid picture of the complex British-Indian relationship through the personal relationship of three boys. What a problem. What a mess. Will they ever straighten it out?

Love, Sally B.

May 23rd, 1945

Dear Mom and Dad,

… I'm working hard again. I'm still weak, but I'm getting stronger. I still cannot run or lift my legs into a jeep without helping myself lift with my arms. It's a pain! But these really young men on Ward #6 are an inspiration. They are so brave and funny and helpful and uncomplaining. Have three nicknames now, "Skip," "Cricket" and "Mumsey"! There is no need to be very formal. These boys are never disrespectful and are so helpful when they can be.

The other night I went on a blind date with Shirl. Shirl's friend Casey, Charles and I drove around the circle from Tacloban to Abuyog to Dulag to Dagami and back. They let both Shirl and me drive the jeep. It's quite a machine. Then we went for a picnic. We had tenderloin steak, French fries and beans. Not bad. It was fun just to get out and this date was very pleasant.

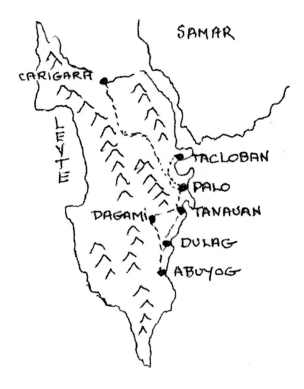

LEYTE ISLAND — 1945

After supper we all drove up to the top of a high hill overlooking Tacloban Harbor. It was a lovely sight, the lovely clouds reflected in the calm water. We heard singing. Behind us, across the hillside was a weaving line of lights, people carrying torches. There was an illuminated cross, stars and lanterns winding around the torturous curves of the path, moving and pulsating to the weird strains of an unfamiliar chant. How strange to us, the two views, the lights of the old city below us and the moving lights of the religious ceremony moving along the hillside. It was lovely.

Junior and Dottie were married last weekend. I had introduced Dottie, one of our group from Devens, to Junior when we went to a party in Hollandia. She is so pretty and was lovely in a dress made of a white parachute. They had a Catholic wedding in the church here in the town where we are, in the old Spanish Cathedral. It was a lovely service. They were given three days off in some general's beach house with a flush john, showers, a Filipino maid and all the fixings one could imagine out here. We are all very happy for them.

Well, I've finally gotten some pina cloth for you. It is a delicate cloth made of pineapple-leaf fibers, which can be made into tablecloths. The other piece is abaca; a courser cloth made of coconut fibers. I have acquired another pair of sandals. These fit. But goods here are going up in price.

Oh, and two nights ago we had a terrific earthquake. Everyone woke up. It lasted about 45 seconds, followed by two more tremors. I was excited. This was my second one over here. We had one in New Guinea, too.

Oh my goodness, I almost left out the most important part. Cousin Eunice's husband Everett called on me last week!! We talked for about two hours and he showed me pictures of his kids and Cousin Eleanor's daughter. Remember that we had never met. I was in nursing school when Eunice was married and unable to leave school. It was a funny but nice way to meet one's cousin-in-law. He was very nice. Nice to catch up on the family!

Love, Me

May 31, 1945

Dear Folks,

… Forgive the lull in letters. I've been tired when I get off work. Still can't run, but I'm getting stronger. Now Shirl, Betty and Mickey are in the hospital with the amoeba! What a drag. I do feel for them. BC and I are holding down the fort.

I've been working awfully hard this week. Hard as it is, it is a joy to work with these very young soldiers. We all do a lot of laughing. The ones who can be up, help me with those who are bed patients. I have a lot of baths to give and beds to make and there is so much cooperation there that the work gets done. We have a very happy ward. When these guys get shipped home or back to duty, I know I won't see them again, but I feel as if I have lost some real friends.

I just found out that because there is so much amoebic dysentery here, the colonel is going to give all of us nurses physical exams. He threatened to readmit me because I am so anemic and I weigh so little, but since the transfusion, I'm better and I'm gaining weight. But amoeba are no joke, there is so much here!!

Love, Sally B.

June 3, 1945

Dear Mom and Dad,

Imagine! The sky is falling. We are one of the hospitals on the Base with unlimited late leaves. No more midnight curfew! Anytime up to 6 a.m. is fine as long as we sign in by then!! Can you believe this??

And we now have a lovely lounge tent with a rug, several tables, lounge chairs and couches covered with PINK cloth. There is a stove, bread, cheese, and coffee and eats. It's WONDERFUL. We have much to thank Major McKay for.

We've become, here in the 126th, like a big family. We are all congenial, the nurses, the doctors, the special service people, all the enlisted men. We have all worked and do work so hard! This facility is actually so well cared for and well run, we're like a village. And you know I'm so happy working on this ward.

Last night BC and I read "The Prophet" by Kahlil Gibran. What wonderful philosophies of life he presents, Love, Friendship, Homes, Children, Life, Death. It's beautiful and it makes one feel detached from our real world and work. 'Twould be so wonderful to be able to express one's feelings so well in words. Not many of us can.

From "The Prophet" by Kahlil Gibran

On Friendship
"Your friend is your needs answered.
He is your field which you sow with love and
reap with thanksgiving.
He is your board and your fireside.
For you come to him with your hunger,
And you seek him for peace.

When your friend speaks his mind, you
fear not the 'nay' in your own mind, nor do
you withhold the 'ay.'
And when he is silent your heart ceases
not to listen to his heart;
For without words, in friendship, all
thoughts, all desires, all expectations are
born and shared, with joy that is
unacclaimed.
When you part from your friend, you
grieve not;
For that which you love
most in him may be clearer in his
absence, as the mountain to the
climber is clearer from the plain.
And let there be no purpose in friendship save the dispensing of the spirit.
For love that seeks aught but the dis-
closure of its own mystery is not love but
a net cast forth: and only the unprofitable
is caught.

And let your best be for your friend.
If he must know the ebb of your tide,
let him know its flood also.

175

For what is your friend that you should

seek him with hours to kill?

Seek him always with hours to live.

For it is his to fill your need, not your

emptiness.

And in the sweetness of friendship, let

there be laughter and sharing of pleasures.

For in the dew of little things the heart

finds its morning and is refreshed."[21]

What a beautiful passage. One to keep and to remember.

Love, Sally B.

June 8, 1945

Dear Mom and Dad,

… How amazed and ashamed I am when I realize so many days have passed since I last wrote. I think of you often, picturing you in the garden that I loved, mowing the lawn or entertaining friends, walking through the long soft grass looking for the wild strawberries. I can't believe I was doing that just a year ago. On June 21st I gave all that up temporarily and rode with a beating heart on that stuffy train to Fort Devens. I've been 10 months overseas. These months have been SO full, knowing people, men and women, learning to sort out one's real friends from those who "pass in the night." Best of all I'm doing what I wanted to do, my goal in coming into the Army. I'm helping so many heal their injuries.

[21] From "The Prophet." Kahlil Gibran. Alfred A Knopf, Inc. A Borzoi Book - 1969 ed. p. 58-59.

These have been happy days. I've been reading, writing, and working hard. We now have a young Filipino girl, Julie, who works in our tent for us. She cleans, washes, irons, and mothers us all. The gals in our tent are very congenial. They are stimulating, well read, full of ideas and thoughts of a new life back home. It's hard to write at night because we always end up in a long discussion, so I've ended up going to the recreation tent to write.

All week I've been very busy at work, the ward is packed. One afternoon I was on alone in a veritable whirl, back rubs, shots of penicillin, so awfully many. My penicillin was kept in the icebox in the next ward, so I went flying between the wards in the rain to get my drugs. I reached into the icebox, filled my hands with bottles then started back. Zoom! I slid, and my whole right side was immersed in mud! I lost my bottles.

I shook myself free from the hole I'd driven into the mud. Amid cheers and whistles from both wards, I rose and straightened my soiled dignity. I began to hunt for my bottles. What a mess! I found them, but how foolish I felt!

One afternoon, I brought my camera and lined the guys on Ward #6 up for a picture. They are such a wonderful bunch. Hope it comes out! (*It did not.*) My favorite ones were evacuated this week. I'm so glad they won't be back here. One of the men who is going home, the one who called me "Mumsey" says he will write to you. He flew home. He's the one whose chest muscles were blown to smithereens, whose dressings were so painful to both of us. And he never made a whimper when I did his dressings. A very special young man.

One afternoon just before many men left, we heard a terrible screaming overhead and a *whomp*. The men yelled, "Get down, we're being shelled!." We pulled everyone we could out of bed and put them under their beds. Then I called the chief nurse. These were OUR shells. Someone had programmed the guns wrong and the 126th had mistakenly became a target! Finally, the shells stopped. We put everyone back to bed. It was scary, but no one was hurt. We all bet someone's face was very, very red!!

Another afternoon, suddenly all the wards were yelling and agitated. The noise got nearer and nearer. Patients in their flapping robes and pajamas were following at a distance a HUGE lizard. I mean huge!

The head was lizard-shaped and 12 inches long, the body and tail 12-plus feet long. The tail was triangular and he was swishing it back and forth. Someone yelled, "Stay in the ward! He'll kill you with that tail if it hits you! He'll go under the ward. Leave him alone!!!" No one knew his name.[22]

Anyway, never before have I seen such an animal. I'll never forget the speed with which he raised himself on his four muscular legs and sped under our elevated ward, then under the next one all the way down to the swamp, at whose highest edge our hospital was built. I haven't seen him again. And I am so glad!!

---

[22] When I got home, I looked up what I thought it might have been. It was a monitor lizard for they do live on Leyte.

Oh, could you send me some more air weight paper, bath powder, Bobbie pins?

Great love to you both, Me

June 10, 1945

Dear Dad,

It's Father's Day, and it crept up on me before I knew it! How I wish I could be home to celebrate this special day with a long talk, to hear your worst curse ("Great Scott!") describing the water in the cellar in that lovely dream house in the country!

Your letters are wonderful and mean so much over here. It keeps the bonds tight even though we're so far apart. It will be some get-together when we are together again.

It's your day, Dad. I hope it is a wonderful one for you.

Much love, Sally

June 10, 1945

Dear Grampus,

What's this about your being sick? I hope it is over soon and you'll be back with your own rare spirits. I hope this set back is a short one, Grampus. Even though I'm not there with you, I'm there in spirit, so I'm sending special wishes for a Special Granddad Day on Father's Day.

About a year ago, you and I had that wonderful talk, the one where I aired my doubts and fears about the young friends in the European theater. Those talks were so special to me. It helped me so much in focusing on what I want for my life, a home, a family, a husband who is fine, sensitive, thoughtful, understanding, humorous, who loves people and who has vision. I've met many men here, but nothing is normal, so this is not the place or the time to have time to form deep bonds.

Can't wait to have more good talks with you like we always do. It's late now, but I want to wish you God's speed in getting well and much love on Grandfather's Day.

Your devoted and loving, Sally

June 14, 1945

Dear Mom and Dad,

… I just got your letter about Grampus. It was a real blow because I had no idea it would come to this, but it was a blessing he went so fast. On Sunday, Father's Day, I wrote a long letter to him hoping he'd be better soon. When I was done, I turned to BC and told her I hoped Grampus would get that letter. He never will, but I loved him and he'll know.

I got the letter while I was on duty. "Brooklyn," one of my favorite 19-year-olds, knew something was wrong. He came and sat with me until I was composed. He is so sweet. He brought me a can of rubbing talcum and told me to powder my nose before going out to pass my medicines.

We will all miss Gramps' wonderful appreciation of little things and of the human spirit. But now he's free of his illness and he's with Gram and his earthly worries are over.

Thank you for the lovely way you told me, Mom and Dad. I did love Grampus. His faith in me made me so humble. God bless him in his new and rightful rest. He deserved this final peace with Grandma at last.

Much love, Sally

I recall —

On the ward one event occurred which I will never forget. For some reason, I did not write home about it, but it is still so vivid.

We ran out of penicillin in my ward.

There was a great demand for penicillin, the only antibiotic available at that time. We gave it every three or four hours in an aqueous solution. One of my patients had a gangrene infection in his leg. Already he'd had to have part of his leg below his knee amputated. Still the infection spread. We fought to save his leg above the knee. We ran short of penicillin. We cut doses on all other patients, first on my floor, then the whole hospital, and tried to borrow from other hospitals. Everyone was short because of a longshoreman's strike on the West Coast.

I don't remember ever being so angry, as our hospital cut every dose we could, on everyone we could. We borrowed all over the island to get enough to contain this horrible infection from involving his whole upper thigh, then his body.

We curtailed that infection long enough to board him for home. Eventually we got our penicillin. I will remember those strikers who we felt were so selfish, who were home, who were not putting up with bullets, filth, heat, bugs and all the other joys of the jungle, who were not facing loss of a leg, a thigh and eventual death for lack of this miracle drug all because it was being held up by a strike.

I remember how willing our hospital and others were to go without, to share in this true emergency fight. It became everyone's battle. And he won. He got well. We were all told later that he did get well. We were all so glad.

Penicillin was the only antibiotic we had to use in WWII. It was truly a miracle drug.

Until 1942, while I was still in nursing school, we gave sulfa drugs — sulfadiazine, sulfathiazole and sulfamerazine. These were better than nothing. In 1942 while I was taking Communicable Disease Medicine with Dr. Marion Leonard at Yale, she told us about a woman in isolation who was dying of a streptococcal infection following the birth of her baby. She did not respond to any of the sulfas. She had a hysterectomy, but the fever continued to be dangerously high.

Her husband gave permission for Yale to use an experimental drug — penicillin. It arrived from New York City and was given to the woman.

Dr. Leonard had kept us posted day-by-day on the case. At the opening of class that next morning, she was smiling. "The patient was given penicillin yesterday. This morning her temperature is almost normal! She will live!" This was how I first learned about penicillin.

Head Nurse — Dermatology, Ward #4

June 22, 1945

Dear Mom and Dad,

... Last week, a week ago, I was changed on duty again. My heart broke when I had to leave my boys on Ward #6. I loved them all, so young, so brave. We had so many laughs, despite all the pain and discomfort.

I was sent to be Head Nurse on Ward #4 that is a skin ward. I'm afraid this service is all Greek to me. I have had almost NO dermatology training, but I found there was a GREAT NEED for reorganization. I sent back to the pharmacy fifteen jars of 5% ammoniated mercury and ten of boric acid the other day. Then I got us an icebox, a new sink, new treatment carriages, and a new bulletin board. How the guys kid me, even though I don't know beans, not BEANS about skin. But the doctor officer is willing to teach me as we make rounds and I'm absorbing knowledge like a blotter.

Now we have 60 yards of burlap that will enclose our treatment rooms. There really was a lot to tend to here and it is fun changing things around so things work better. These guys are so nice too, as is my ward officer, so it's not too bad, just not the same as Ward #6. Some of my old patients came to see me on Ward #4 and took me to the movies the other night, "special friends."

Love, Me

Trip to the Old Fort

June 25, 1945

Dear Mom and Dad,

… Haven't been feeling too well. I'm told I have a lot of mending to do, but one afternoon this week on my afternoon off, BC, Jerry D., Dick J. and I climbed up to a Spanish tower about ten miles down the coast from here. It was a very short steep climb. Jerry, a Navy man BC likes, took lots of pictures. What a view from the top. Jerry has a little dog named Digger. He loves him. Digger came along too!

The tower is an old fort, a square structure, we think made of coral blocks. It's gray and there is a tree growing inside. There were long, narrow openings in the original structure, but now there are shell holes in its sides. These openings gleamed white next to the gray walls.

There was a phenomenal view of the harbor and coast. No wonder the fort was built on this hilltop by the Spanish, and no doubt used by the Nips and by us. A real lookout. Many of our ships were in the sea below.

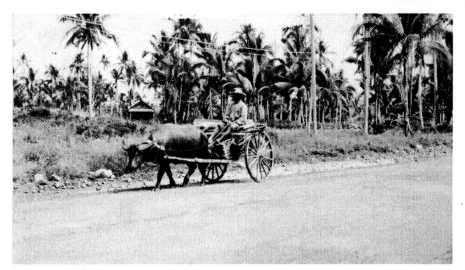

A trip to market

It had been fun. We all ran down. We went to Dick's place for a fried chicken supper. Dick took pictures of the Filipino homes near the road — so primitive. Such a contrast between the carabao pulling a two-wheeled wagon next to speeding Army vehicles. There is a real contrast in life-styles here. I'm told Leyte is very backward compared to many other islands, especially Luzon!

Love, Sally B.

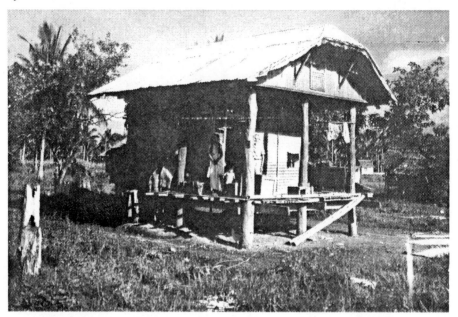

A typical home

June 29, 1945

Dearest Mom and Dad,

… Time is flying by. Another week has passed. Brother John is a year older today—he's 28. Tomorrow is your 29th wedding anniversary. Congratulations to all of you.

This has been my week of reconstruction. Ward #4 has been functioning for six months with a mere minimum. This week, with all that burlap, we made the treatment rooms, a doctor's office, and an examining room. The drugs are organized a la Major McKay and our icebox is a godsend.

There are many soaks and dressings to do so I am VERY busy. Doctors make rounds, so I go with them and take new orders.

Well, guess what?! Ward #4 has never passed inspection before. We, and two other wards, won a beer allotment for the ward Saturday. We were all tickled pink because all the guys and I worked so hard remodeling the ward.

Love, Sally

July through September
Transfer to Orthopedics, Ward #24

July 2, 1945

Dear Folks,

Sunday I was moved again!!! This time I know I left the ward in better shape than when I went there. I'm on Ward #24, Orthopedics!! So, I'm in the ward now which pleases me! I love to work with "contraptions" because the nurse can do so much to help those patients locked into casts.

Several times last week we all went swimming. We drove first down the coast to Dulag past the cemetery where there were acres of white crosses — our men, with one dog tag on the cross for identification. The cemetery was green and closely cut around the acres of evenly spaced crosses. Our flag whipped in the breeze, blowing over this area surrounded by a white picket fence. It was a peaceful place. But what a loss! I was moved to tears. So many, so young, so far from home!

Then we went to a deserted airstrip where we saw some wrecked Jap planes and some of our functional ones. Driving back to the beach, we saw a sight to behold. A woman walked along the road dressed in a colored shirt and a skirt of parachute silk and a big bunch of bananas on her head! Like Carmen Miranda!!

Swimming was fun, jumping, laughing, and diving to the bottom. My date was a young man who is in charge of convalescent training. It was such a relaxing time. He loves to talk and I have just plain fun with him.

Another night, Carl took me to watch him develop some pictures he took of Filipino life. It was fun to have a lesson in how to develop and print film. Carl has given me some great prints to keep since I have so few films for my camera. I have some good pictures of here, but very few in Hollandia, which was so beautiful.

I've been quiet for a few days. Had cholera and typhoid updates. They always make me sick.

I can just imagine the house now in July, all cool and shady with your lovely thriving garden of vegetables and flowers. It's a vivid memory I keep until I sail into the yard again with a yell to greet you both!

By the way, did I tell you I now have a Philippine Ribbon, an Asiatic Ribbon with two combat stars, and two overseas stripes? This all means 34 points!

Give my love to the neighbors. I like to think of all of you and your breezes. It's so terribly hot here!!

Love, Sally B.

July 7, 1945

Dear Mom and Dad,

… Spring at home sounds almost as wet as it was dry here. What a shame about the hay again this year. It was poor last year because it was so dry, now it's spoiled this year because it is so wet! Imagine the hardships early farmers must have had with no reserves or stores to fall back on!!

I want to tell you about yesterday. It was a wonderful day, my long day for July! I slept late, for me, it was 9:00 a.m. Shirl got up at 10:00. We went into the lounge tent and made scrambled eggs, bananas, toast and coffee. Shirl and Betty and I sat and talked for hours about the war, its ending someday, and the children who will be born into the post-war world. We all felt grateful in a way that we will have understanding of the pain and anguish our men have had to face in fighting this war. We all felt that people must know what a cost war exacts. We all must teach and work for a better solution to national and international problems.

In the afternoon, Carl, Casey, Shirl and I went for a ride, a wonderful ride in the rain. We went way down the coast to a little fishing village, drove around and ended up in a charming old cathedral. It was very old. We went into the dimly lighted nave. Light came through the stained glass window. It was beautiful, so quiet, so peaceful. A priest came in and we asked him how old the church was. He said it was 140 years old. He was so nice.

When I got home that night, I had a letter from Dan. He had been enroute home to Michigan for three months but he was back home at last, sending in orders for milk, ice cream, steaks, green salads and a bath. He'd been in a cast for weeks. He was having a whirl. How glad his family was to have him home! He did not lose his arm!

I finished "American Guerrilla in the Philippines." Thanks for the book, I loved it. Some of the action takes place right near here. Then I got a box of books from brother John. This will keep me out of mischief!!

I'm enjoying orthopedics. It's a challenge taking care of these guys in pulleys, weights and casts. I'm glad I'm trained to make a difference in their stay here. I'm so glad I'm a nurse. It is a very satisfying way to build and not to destroy in this war.

Love, Me

Promotion to 1st Lieutenant

July 14, 1945

Dear Folks,

… A most extraordinary thing happened to me this morning. I was working hard when I was called to the Chief Nurse's office.

"Am I to be moved again?" I wondered. "I seem to stay put such a short time! What have I done now? Have I broken some Army regulation?"

So, I went to Major McKay's office, very nervous indeed. One did not get called in without a reason!

"Did Major McKay want to see me?" I asked in the front office.

"Just wait a minute outside, please," her assistant said. So, I stood outside. I was surer and surer I must have done something awful! Then Miss McKay came out and told me to come in her office where the hospital's Colonel Dismukes and the two assistant chief nurses were waiting. Then the colonel said some very nice things and read a statement stating that as of July 6th, I was promoted to 1st Lt. ANC.

"Dear Lt. Hitchcock,

Congratulations on your promotion to First Lieutenant! It is a pleasure to have this opportunity to personally express to you my heartfelt congratulations and thanks for a job well done.

Your conscientious work has merited this promotion and is greatly appreciated by myself and your commanding officer.

I am confident you will continue to serve your country to the best of your ability and with renewed vigor, apply yourself faithfully to the task that lies ahead.

Sincerely,

E. Jeff Barnette

Col. CAC Commanding"

I was speechless, red-faced, and wordless. I was completely taken aback and unprepared as Miss McKay pinned on my silver bar. I'm afraid I was not very gracious. I think someone asked me if I wanted to say "Thanks." I believe I did, then I left to go back to work. The first thing that was said was, "Oh, ho, she's got a promotion!" I've been in a year.

Well, Dad, how about mailing me your 1st Lt. bars?! I can't wear my gold ones anymore. I'd be proud to wear yours!! (*My father's were for the Spanish-American War and inappropriate, so I had to buy current ones.*)

When I went back on the floor, the guys were so cute. One from surgery came over and said, "This is one promotion I'm really happy about, Sally. I'm so glad!" Many hand shakes all around. It really was no big deal because I had been in a year and soon all would get their promotions too.

In the afternoon, two of my favorite banged-up patients left for home. How glad I was for them. After work, I went back to write letters home for two men in arm casts. One had not told his family how badly he was hurt, so he asked me to tell them. It was a challenge to tell the truth about his state of health, and not scare them. Sam is a wonderful guy who has a lot of injuries. The first time I did his dressings, I almost was sick like when I did that Navy boy with the knee in Hollandia. But I was not sick and he's so spunky. Never a whimper. I am in awe of their fortitude!!

Love, 1st Lt. Sally B.

July 23, 1945

Dear Mom and Dad,

… So glad you got the tablecloths I sent! Two days ago I got a box from you mailed last FALL!! Had yarn, stationary, lipstick and bobby pins. The package was rewrapped and sent through Biak Island. I have gotten the two books you sent, "Pastoral" and "Cluny Brown." Never have enough to read so I do thank you for your thoughtfulness!

I'm so surprised to hear brother John is back in England. I'm glad, for sitting in the Florida Keys was not to his liking at all!!

Oh well, the big news is I'm to go on nights again. Every time I go on nights something momentous happens. I'm quite a fatalist now. I've never ever completed a full night duty.

#1   We left Fort Devens for overseas

#2   We left for the Philippines

#3   I got amoeba

#4   Who knows?

Today one of my patients gave me a guitar handmade in Cebu, another island in the Philippines. He's such a sweet guy on his way home. He's a front line medic and he's seen so much. I admire these guys. They deserve a lot of credit for saving so many lives!!

Whew, the mosquitoes are awful tonight! The weather is HOT and sticky with rain each day. Guess the dry season is ending. Speaking of rain, I hear there is a flood at home. Tell me all! …

Love, Sally B.

July 29, 1945

Dear Folks,

… Just before night duty, I had to go through a battery of tests again because of continuing fatigue and symptoms. The doctor said that if they found ulcerations he'd send me home!! But all is well. No ulcerations, negative exam, so I'm to REST! And I go on nights.

Last week, Shirl, Casey, Carl and I had a wonderful afternoon swimming at the beach, followed by a picnic. It was a lot of fun. We are all good friends.

Major McKay and eight girls have left for home. I'm sorry to see her go, but glad for her. Slowly the world changes here. More and more people are leaving. The war progresses. The Philippines are secured. I hope I will get home soon, but not on sick leave and I'm sure I won't this time.

Miss McKay was a corking good chief nurse, with high standards and fair. We will all miss her level hand. She made a terrific unit out of the 126th! Now we will have either or both of the assistant chiefs, Captain Radacovich or Captain Burkwall, as our new chief.

Love, Sally B.

August 2, 1945

Dear Mom and Dad.

… People are starting to discuss life after the war. It's strange to know that somewhere in the future, this terrible war will be over out here, too.

I talked with a group of gals and with a radar officer about his dream for the future. He talks and collects ideas from people over here in different professions. What he dreams of doing is to get a group of young, ambitious, congenial people to form a corporation backed by interests in the States. If he can get $100,000 stateside backing and secure discarded heavy Army equipment for land and sea work over here, he'd set up a plan to utilize the vast mineral reserves as well as oil, mahogany, teak and pineapples. Then he'd send them to the States, where after the war, the market will be bottomless.

After the money and work bring returns, then comes the social movement. This interests me. He plans an ideal community with schools for the children, ideal housing, socialized medicine, public health and medical research. What a wonderful dream. A lot of the staff here are interested. Manila would be within easy reach by air. What a dream. It might be fun when all this war is over!

Many of the fliers see a real future in air service and many of us begin to wonder what will be at home for us when we return. Maybe brother John might be interested. I've sent this prospectus to Dan. I wonder about my future at home. I had no stateside nursing experience, a lot of varied Army experience. Will there be a job for me when I get home?

Shirl and Betty are back in the hospital. What an unhealthy crew! But at least we have been told the 126th will not move. It is to be a permanent base hospital, an ideal spot, beautifully landscaped.

Brother John is ferrying B-17s home from England now. I was surprised because he tried to get out here. I'm glad it's all over in England. Last time he was in London was during the Robot Blitz.

Love, Sally B.

August 7, 1945

Dear Folks,

… It's my third night on nights, Wards #1, #2, #3, #4, two skin and two medical wards. My first two nights were very busy, some mighty sick men. Sometimes the Army makes me very angry. For two nights I raised rim to the MD about one patient and for two nights the MD kept saying, "We can't do anything tonight."

When the day crew came on at the end of the second night, I raised the roof. And action took place — an operation for an intestinal obstruction!

… Nights is not too bad this time. The four ward men are hard workers and after the first couple of nights, I'm not too busy …

Love, Me

The War is Over

August 14, 1945

Dear Mom and Dad,

… For the past few days I've been dying to write you — THAT IT'S ALL OVER, that this terrible war has ended and what it was like over here when word first came over the radio. My wards were bedlam. What a time! I wouldn't have missed it for anything, being on nights, that first night when the news of the surrender came over.

My four wards went wild. I have never been hugged or kissed or spun around so many times in my whole life. Even had a dance with a cute young guy who had been over here 28 months and states that this was his first dance in all that time! How wonderful it was to see such pure, unadulterated joy and bedlam, and real smiles and laughter!! Of course each night my ward men and I were sweating out the news, ready at the moment to switch on the lights and say it is all over. AN EVENT TO REMEMBER!

Just before I went on nights for the fourth time, I told the kids it was my luck in the Army to have something momentous happen. It did! There was the surrender. Then I went to bed, slept and did not know until late this afternoon. Plunged into bed this morning and slept all day, staggered into the tent at 4:30 p.m. from the night nurses' quarters.

"Anything happen today?" I asked.

"Oh nothing new! Of course you knew the war was over!"

That's how I knew. What a momentous event!!

I think back to the news we got of the dropping of the atomic bomb. First we were ecstatic, then there was this reaction to the reality of its awesomeness. There were endless discussions about what had happened, joy, guilt, thoughtfulness. What a gamut of emotions. Above all was the relief we would not have to invade Japan. We all knew there would have been terrible casualties if we had to invade.

And so it's over. Now the talk is how and when we will get home. Maybe for Christmas — "I'm Dreaming of a White Christmas" and "When the Lights Go On Again All Over the World." How appropriate these song titles are now. Some homes will be so happy this year — not just because it's Christmas, but knowing there will not be a dreaded telegram at the door!

Before I close, I have to tell you about a very nice experience. It's been nine months since I slept in a real bed in my tent except for the first week when we came here. We've been on canvas cots. Tomorrow we get *real beds* again which we gave up to the patients when our hospital was so overcrowded. So, back to civilization!

Love, Me!

August 23, 1945

Dear Mom and Dad,

So many history-making events have taken place since I last wrote to you! And I have completed ONE WHOLE NIGHT DUTY! That was a victory after one whole year of trying.

You can imagine the rumors that are flying around since the end of the war — all about getting home. This is number one on everyone's mind, to begin life again. Every angle is discussed by everyone and no one knows any more today than they ever did, except the soldiers will be going home sooner than any of us dreamed possible. It's too soon to know, but we all dream and speculate!

I'm on another skin ward. My ward officer is so pleasant, sympathetic and fine. He's a ship platoon doctor on detached service with us. And I'm learning. He likes to teach and I am lapping up everything he says and enjoying stretching my mind. There is lots to learn about skin problems out here with the heat, fungus, bacteria, lack of cleanliness. It all causes problems. I should know first hand!!

You can well imagine the mood out here now. It is an atmosphere of suspended animation, really suspended. Excitement! Everyone is full of thoughts and dreams about home, hopes and prayers, and endless discussions of points and points and points. Me, I have only 36 points, so every time I hear these guys with 100s, I feel foolish to mention home. I want to get home so badly; I'd row if I had a chance.

Speaking of rumors, the whole hospital was alerted that the colonel was going to make a speech of great importance at noon to the officers, at night to the detachment. Needless to say, I went with the rest, a group running madly to lunch. There was NO speech at all. That's how strong rumors are. We all expect this unit to break up soon, but we don't know.

To top it all, (I guess to keep the lid on) we have become very GI. Starting this morning all enlisted personnel, officers and nurses arose at 5:30 a.m. to stand reveille — fully clothed!! Shirl is a platoon leader. All this brought on a frenzy of gripes, anger! The notice stated, "To lower the V.D. rate, boost morale and promote military courtesy!" Well, we raised many quiet questions, but we did what we were told.

And thanks, Dad, for my three sets of silver bars; I needed them for my collars. I really need them now for the "spit and polish" attitude here since Major McKay left.

We were the saddest sacks when we staggered to the area this morning, slumped to attention, and gradually woke up enough to know we had a whole half hour to watch the sun rise before we went to chow.

Up to now, we have been very relaxed with each other, a very conscientious, hard-working unit who knew each other well. Now we must salute officers of greater rank and be very proper Army personnel. I suppose this must be to keep discipline when everyone is SO ecstatic!!

Last night I had a date with a P-38 pilot. He has 112 points!! He joined the RAF first, then our AAF. He was in England until two years ago, flying Wellingtons. BC and Don, Dodie and her date and my pilot and I went swimming. It was so pleasant. Then we went riding along the beach in the jeep.

"Stop," I called. "I saw some crabs!"

Thousands of little crabs were running towards the water — little white ones. It was beautiful. The moon was full and the ocean pure silver and these little white crabs seemed like tiny moonbeams running into the quiet waters of the sea. Every now and then something so lovely makes a deep impression. This lovely experience was memorable.

Betty's birthday is Sunday, my long day for August. She'll be discharged from the hospital Saturday, so BC and I have arranged for a cake and Shirl and Mickey for ice cream. So, we'll really celebrate! Last year we were at Camp Stoneman in a frenzy of excitement, getting ready to leave for points unknown. This will be a real celebration for her.

Love, Sally B.

August 28, 1945

Dear Folks,

… Life goes on. There is less work for all of us. Carl left for home two days ago. He was consistently a good friend and took my buddies and me around the island many times. Always a gentleman, I hope he can repair his marriage. So many sad disruptions over here.

Guess what! I wore a dress the other night, the first time in a year! Orders came out we can wear dresses after duty. We all flew to our footlockers and delved deep into the moldy smelling footlockers and retrieved our dresses. My beige dress is ruined, stained all brown in the front. My dark one is wearable because I can't see the stains. It will seem strange to blossom out in a dress, stockings and shoes, not high Army lace-ups and wool socks! Guess mosquito control is effective!!

Of course, the dress deal came down soon after the reveille order.

Went to Dick's quarters to meet Casey and Shirl before a dance. I was shocked. His is a segregated quarter master unit. I was not aware of whole units of Negro men and it came as a shock. No wonder I never saw any Negroes in my hospital. I was overwhelmed with a feeling of terrible guilt and unease. I was glad when we left. It was not a good feeling. It is wrong!!

Love, Sally B.

August 31, 1945

Dear Mom and Dad,

... Such a week of excitement. Shirl and I got our orders to move to a new unit, the 73rd Field Hospital, which we are told may go to Japan in the Army of Occupation. The sad thing is BC, Betty and Mickey will not go with us, but we'll be nearby for a while. I'll have to send you a new APO.

The other exciting event was that I was advised to have my last lower wisdom tooth extracted before I left this unit, so I did on the 28th. It was not pleasant! It took over an hour and a half for that dentist to get it out, hacking, drilling and chiseling. As a result, I developed cellulitis and my face is a straight line from my ear to my shoulder and I'm back in the hospital on penicillin, hot and cold packs, codeine. It will pass.

Right opposite me in bed is a nurse friend who came here actively ill from a scorpion bite on her derriere as she sat on the john. She went into anaphylactic shock reaction, swelled up all over, could hardly breathe. She's better now, but that was scary.

I guess I am glad to look forward to a new adventure in a different climate, but it is hard to leave this unit, of which we were such an integral part. We have so many friends. It has become our home. Guess we're going to Kyushu, a southern Japanese island, near where Uncle Ed was.

Word has spread that we are leaving. Many people all over the hospital in all ranks have expressed sorrow that we are going. I'm sorry, sorry because I've worked so hard here caring for the women who served and the guys hurt on Leyte, Luzon, and all the other liberated islands. I've made many friends, but one-by-one these units will change as the needs change.

Love, Sally B.

Accolades to the 126th General

A quote from the
"Sauna News"

Anniversary Issue   Friday, 21 September 1945

"General Eichelberger Tells the 126th

Praise for its service to the Eighth Army came to the 126th General Hospital yesterday in a formal commendation from Lt. Gen. R. L. Eichelberger, Commanding General of the Eighth Army.

... Gen. Eichelberger's commendation dated August 10, 1945, came to Col. J.B. Dismukes, 126th Commanding Officer on an ornamental page suitable for framing. The general wrote, "It affords me great pleasure to express to the officers and men of the 126th General Hospital, my personal appreciation for the wholehearted and enthusiastic cooperation which you have given the Eighth Army in the conduct of the Southern Philippines Operations. The long hours and hard work which you put into the treatment and care of casualties should be repaid at least in part, by the knowledge that your work has saved many lives and lessened the suffering of many wounded men. The fine record of your unit reflects great credit on you and the United States Army."

Further endorsement came from Base K Headquarters Col. E.G. Itsherer, Major Gen. Evart G. Plank and Lt. General Styer.

(A short history finalized these tributes for which we received the Meritorious Award — a badge featuring a wreath to be sewn onto our uniform sleeve).

For this Anniversary Issue, Col. J.B. Dismukes writes:

"... As you all remember we arrived in the Philippines as a 1500-bed hospital. At first glance our hospital looked desolate and the idea of setting up an installation at first seemed impossible. But each member worked day and night in spite of constant rain, mud, enemy aerial activity and almost every discomfort imaginable. Through such individual contributions, there was established a 2750 bed hospital which in eight months of operation has cared for more than 27,000 ward patients and many other thousands in its clinics.

The hospital has been visited and inspected by many high-ranking officials including the Surgeon General. Each has been profuse in his praise of what has been accomplished here.

Each one of you can now look around and see your own handiwork and be proud that you have built and operated a hospital second to none in the Pacific — or the ETO. Your own ideas and suggestions, your loyalty and your hard work have made your contribution to the war one to be envied and admired.

Whatever my future, I will always consider being the commanding officer of the 126th General Hospital my greatest honor and privilege.

J.B. Dismukes, Col." [23]

September 12, 1945

Dear Mom and Dad,

... We know you haven't gotten our mail for ages, because it's still sitting in the PO waiting for planes and ships to take it out. And we've not gotten mail for days. I've had two letters from you since V-J Day, dated August 11 and 27.

The trip to Japan in the Army of Occupation is not far off. Shirl and I have sent emergency orders for heavy underwear, heavy lined pants, jackets, vests, gloves, hats and overshoes. So, I guess it's going

[23] Ibid p. 3, 4, "Sauna News"

to be cold. Guess we'll feel the change since we're so acclimated to this equatorial climate now.

I'm sending home a large box of books, the guitar from Cebu and four bolo knives. The knives are for you and Dad, John and Dan. The shells from Leyte are for me.

I'm sending it September 13th. I did receive the inner lining of my coat that you sent and my dress suits and a large tube of toothpaste. Thank you so much. Seems funny to be thinking of cold weather. With all the cold weather gear we are compiling, I'm sure it will be very cold where we are going.

Still no word about moving from the 126th, but I'm sure it will be soon. The rains have begun again. It is very muddy like it was when we first came here.

Monday night was a night I'll not soon forget.

Duffy, Johnny, Shirl and I had cooked steaks and onions over the Coleman stove in our tent. We were full and happy and had dishes to do. So, we turned on the radio. Our lights went out. The next tent had dim lights, then we smelled burning wires. We ran for the guard to pull the switch for the area lights but he didn't know where the switch was. A nurse knew and pulled it in the nick of time for as I tore back, the tent next to us, BC's tent, was on fire. We grabbed blankets and got it out before it had gone too far and long before the firemen got there. Guess we saved the nurses' area!!

After the fire, I went up to the club and played gin with my ward officer who was leaving for home and to his wife and three kids, the next day. He's the one who belonged to a ship platoon and with whom I worked on the skin ward. He beat me alive but we both had a nice evening.

Next item. The nurses here have been given permission to fly to a dance on the island of Cebu. Guess the powers-that-be are trying to bolster our morale. I hear the guys on Cebu need their morale bolstered too. We're told it will be 45 minutes by air. It should be fun and a real change and a chance to fly over some of the other islands we've been hearing about.

Love, Sally B.

The 77th Division Dance at Cebu

September 18, 1945

Dear Folks,

… I have so much to tell you this time, it's hard to know where to begin. First of all, nurses with 35 points can go home. I have 37, so whenever the ball begins to roll, I'll be on the list, so don't send any Christmas packages. I'll pick them up when I get home! Imagine!!

The second thing this week was the trip to Cebu. I don't know why the powers-that-be gave the nurses a break, but they did and we've all been flown over to the 77th Division Dance. Shirl and I went Saturday afternoon in a PBY (*a flying shore patrol Navy plane with pontoons*) like John flew at first. It was a wonderful trip over and back. I flew the plane for about five minutes, as did others who wanted to (with much help!) How lovely the islands look from the air.

When we landed there were rows and rows of jeeps to pick us up. We were driven in convoys around the outskirts of Cebu City about 20 miles down the coast to the 77th Division. Such different country here. There are hills and trees looking like oaks, fewer palms and cleaner, taller people and cement highways!

All the nurses were housed in the guesthouse, a Spanish-type house with polished floors and tall, blue-painted walls. It was the strangest and most delightful feeling to be within real walls in a real house!! It was the first house since I left home, June 21, 1944. There were flush johns, real sinks. It was really civilized!! When we got ready, we were all transported to the dance area. I met General Bruce and thanked him for arranging this party. I told him also how exciting it was to get off the island of Leyte where we had been for nine months. Leyte is backward and simple compared to Luzon and now I know, Cebu. He was charming.

We were lined up and were observed by the male officers across the room. It was quite like dancing school (long ago) when the boys on one side chose girls on the other side. We all felt rather defenseless.

Gradually we were all chosen. My date was 37 and very pleasant. Eventually, we were escorted to the 77th Division Headquarters Dance.

It was a pretty rowdy party. The wine flowed freely. Seems it was one of the first dances these guys had had in a long time. I had a good time talking to my date, and I learned that Cebu was a center for a leper colony. The Japanese had let everyone out. Who knows what has happened to them, poor souls. Hope they will get treatment.

I was taken home by midnight and tried to sleep. There were NO mosquito nets. Between fighting bugs, trying to keep cool and being kept awake by the gals coming in all night in shifts, I didn't sleep much. I got up early Sunday morning to a delicious meal, real oranges and pears. Had almost forgotten what fresh oranges and pears taste like.

At 8:30 a.m. the jeep convoy picked us up and headed for the airstrip, back into our PBY, and on to Leyte. It had been a wonderful trip, across the mountains where Carl had driven me to Carigara back in April. The ocean reefs were a heavenly aquamarine color. It was a wonderful treat just to get away, to have a change of scene. All a morale builder for the guys and gals as we all wait to go home.

For the last two days I've just slept when I was off. I don't know why I'm so tired, my bounce seems to be gone. At any rate, I've slept much better than I have for several months. Maybe it's the real mattress on a real bed, maybe just the change we had in Cebu. Maybe all the hard work with so little time off is really catching up because it's been a long time since any of us had a real rest. One long day a month since May, a half day a week since March — that's all. From January through March we had no time off. We took care of SO many sick and wounded guys. It was worth it, but maybe all these hours are catching up!!

Another thing that happened last week. The 126th had a seven and one-half pound baby boy, Mike Saunders, son of an Army lieutenant and a Spanish girl. She's darling. I knew her when she was a patient on Ward #25, my Women's Ward. We were all excited. Helen is a charming person and we've all been waiting for Mike!

No word yet on our transfer to the 73rd Field and Japan. We're waiting. I'd like to go, but I'd love to get home …

Love, Sally B.

We move to the 73rd Field Hospital
Army of Occupation

September 24, 1945

Dear Mom and Dad,

… As you can see we have moved at last. It was a very sad day for me to leave the 126th, my home away from home, my buddies, and my friends. It's not easy to pull up stakes, to go somewhere new with all new people, new systems and new surroundings. I had worked so hard at the 126th, seemed to get my real nursing experience there, help build it into the unit it became and, we were told, will now become a permanent base hospital.

Leaving was sad. Everyone was sad to see us go, like leaving home! Shirl and I got a couple of guys to help us move since the hospital did not provide transportation. I'm sure if Major McKay had been there we would not have had to provide our own transportation, but everything is so different now. Everything, everywhere is being cut back and is confused. There are only 1,000 patients left at 126th compared to the 2,892 at our fullest in the spring.

Love, Sally B.

Detached Service
116th Station Hospital

September 26, 1945

Dear Folks,

Our men in the 73rd Field are staging for Japan. We are on temporary duty with the 116th Station Hospital, which has taken over the 73rd Field. We expect to go to Japan about November.

Shirl and I have very nice quarters. We have a pyramidal tent all to ourselves and so much shelf space and furniture we don't know what to do with ourselves. Our tent is screened, a real bed with two mattresses, a desk, a clothes rack and a shelf for shoes. There are several incidental shelves and a large table with a drawer in the middle of the room.

Near our tent is a Red Cross trailer kitchenette where there is always food to cook or snack on. Really, we are more than comfortable and all the other nurses are warm and friendly. Many I knew when they were patients on Ward #25 when I was head nurse, it being the main Women's Ward on the base. Well, here we are and a new chapter begins!

Since now we are not overworked, I've had a few dates with a pleasant captain in the chemical engineering corps Shirl introduced me to. He's married, can't wait to go home, but he's being nice to Shirl and me. Casey, Joe and I have been having fun after hours. He's bright and intellectually stimulating, so off-hours are relaxing.

When Shirl and I arrived yesterday, we unpacked then we walked along the elevated boardwalk to the mess hall which is almost a half-mile from our tent. Our chow is delicious and on plates, on a tablecloth!! What a thrill that was. It's been a long time. The only other times we've eaten in so much style has been with the Navy!

My new address is:

73rd Field Hosp., c/o 116th Sta. Hosp.

APO 1000 c/o PM - San Francisco, Cal.

Love, Me

September 28, 1945

Dear Mom and Dad,

… Today was a day to be remembered! I've been so busy on this medical floor I can hardly see straight. A diphtheria case was admitted to my floor. Of course, there was immediate isolation, then transfer. One young Filipino soldier went sour, had pneumonia and became irrational. There were emergency calls, chest aspirations. Oh dear, I felt so lost because I didn't know where anything was, who to call. It was not my best hour. But we all survived somehow. It does take a breaking-in period to be most effective!

How wonderful to get mail today. Alleluia! I'm so glad John is OUT and you've visited Captain Smith and his wife. He was so good to Shirley and me. Sounds as if you were eye-deep in canning. Well, now John is home, you'll have help. Wish I were there!

We don't know when or if we will move at all. With the war over, there is rumor that only people with low points will go into occupation up north. We will wait and we will be told. What a headache all this reshuffling must be with everyone who can go, chomping at the bit to go home!

Shirl, Casey, Joe and I still make a pleasant foursome. Shirl is about to announce her engagement to Bob, whom she met at Fort Devens, so that when she gets home they will be married. That is so wonderful and happy. Joe will go to Manila soon and Casey home. The old order changeth!

Love, Sally B.

October through November

October 3, 1945

Dear Mom and Dad,

… Everything is in a turmoil. Shirl's and my names have gone in to go home! What a dream. We know now sometime in the near future we'll be on our way. We will NOT go to Japan. We will leave Leyte for San Francisco. We can hardly believe that we are on the list to go, but when?? We know we will not stay here because the 116th is getting new nurses and those of us in the 73rd Field are going home. So, we're in for another move somewhere.

Now the FUTURE really becomes a reality. What will I do when I get home? I'll take a vacation for a few weeks then maybe I'll try Yale or Presbyterian Hospitals, maybe Transoceanic Airlines. I'll have to buckle down to some real thinking soon for the Army is about to end for me, a goal I had for four years. Anyway, I helped a lot in this endeavor and I'm glad.

Time off continues to be pleasant. Our foursome goes to dances. There has been a great effort to supply recreation for so many that wait. We've been sightseeing. We've swum. It's been fun playing bridge and talking. Everyone waits ...

Love, Sally B.

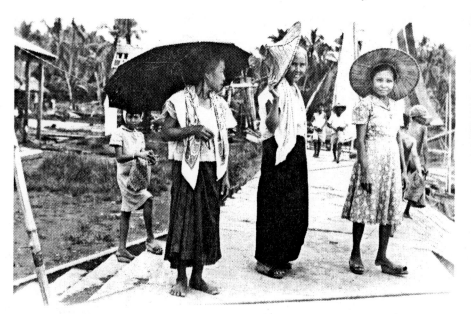

Women at Tanauan.

October 15, 1945

Dear Mom and Dad,

… Work continues. I dream of getting home for a real vacation, rest then relax and then look around for possible places to work. It's funny, scary, to think about shifting gears from the Army where all of us were desperately working towards the same goal, where I was testing my wings in my first job as a graduate nurse and where most of our creature needs were taken care of. Now there is the great void. Many questions arise.

How will it be at home? Will people be glad to see us? Will there be a job for an ex-Army nurse whose main experience has been with gun shot wounds, plastic surgery, skin and tropical medicine? Not too much of that in New England.

We're still on tenterhooks, waiting. It's so hot here now, we're anxious, like everyone else, but the good news is our replacements have come which means one step nearer a ship home. We were told we might be home for Christmas. I don't hope too much! I'll be happy just to be on some old tub headed in the right direction.

Joe and Casey have been sent to Manila so our social life has stopped. Bed early these days. Shirl dreams of her coming wedding. It's fun to hear all her plans.

Yesterday we had a HUGE earthquake! We had just come off duty at 3:30 p.m., and were lying on our beds resting. Suddenly everything in the tent began to tremble. All the pictures on my desk fell down. Our T-bars collapsed. Shirl and I ran outside away from the tent on the wooden platform to the path outside. It was weird. The ground we were standing on was undulating in waves, hills and valleys, dust. We just stood there transfixed. There was no terra firma. Soon it stopped but that was a real one. I've no idea what scale it would measure, but I think it would have done damage to rigid buildings. This was number three for us!

Love, Sally B.

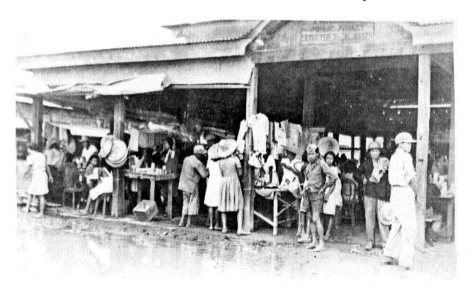

Market at Tanauan.

October 29, 1945

Dear Folks,

… We are still very busy, new replacements or not. It is so hot it is wearing. So working keeps me happy. I'm so glad I'm a nurse. People always get sick, so somehow I'll always be able to find a way to support myself and be happy.

Love, Me

November 2, 1945

Dear Mom and Dad,

... Nice things have happened this week. My old college friend Ted married a French girl in France at Versailles. Sent him congratulations. Then I heard from Dan. It had been a long time since he'd written after he got home.

I wrote him funny letters while he was in the hospital and I was in the hospital too, but he was a long time getting well enough to go home. Now he's home. Seems as though he's working days in commercial art, and going to night school in French, Algebra, Trig, English and Chemistry. What a load! He took entrance exams to the University of Michigan and did so well he will be given two year's credit. Guess he's aiming for pre-med. It's wonderful to hear about a friend whose dreams are finally coming to fruition.

I can't believe it! Shirl just came in. We're being moved again, still on Leyte, but this time to the 44th General. I'm told this hospital is right on the beach! Today too, RFD #2, West Brattleboro, Vermont, was painted on my footlocker, so our time is coming. Our orders will be cut this week. Soon, it's coming, homeward bound!!! ...

Love, Sally B.

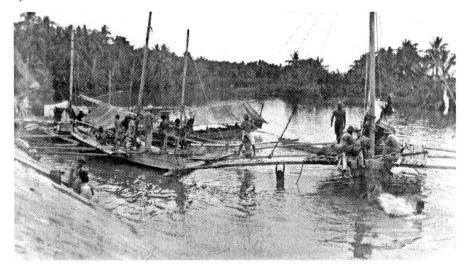

Outriggers at Tanauan

Detached Service
44th General Hospital

November 5, 1945

Dear Mom and Dad,

Here we are at a new APO 1003 PM, San Francisco. Yes, we are right on the beach. It's comfortable but we have NO laundry facilities. We are really busy which is a godsend.

I'm on an officers' medical-surgical floor, and (now I'll tell you a secret), my ward officer told the chief nurse that I'm a wonderful nurse. That was pleasing because I have had those dreadful symptoms again. So, I went to be checked again. Nothing positive, so I'm sure it will all go when I get home. Guess tonight I feel a little down. Waiting is hard.

Love, Me

November 10, 1945

Dear Mom and Dad,

… Hard work is healing. I'm very busy. Got my old nickname back, "Skip." Don't know where it came from, but I'm back in the old swing. Each moment I'm off, I'm on the beach swimming. It's really a dream to put on your suit and walk ten feet and be on the beach. Always before we had to have a male officer or hospital appointed driver take us. Now here we are. I'm so tan you will not know me. By a month from now, I'll be black!!

Shirl and I have had to move to a new tent because our assigned one leaked. We have it to ourselves and enjoy it very much. We iron our shirts on our footlockers and send our pants to the quartermaster's laundry. It's not ideal but nothing is perfect. Hey, Mom, I really iron a snappy shirt now!

It's really nice here, GI and all, but we are cool, so close to the ocean all day and night! We don't even mind the crabs that walk in and out of our tents. They are funny and awkward little fellows.

Love, Sally B.

November 12, 1945

Dear Mom and Dad,

The big news came today! All nurses on Leyte already on orders are leaving tomorrow. All 91 nurses not on orders will be on orders as of tomorrow. That's us. We will leave within a week. We may not make Christmas, but soon thereafter. When we really leave, I'll write to give you the date we leave and the name of the ship so you can check the newspapers for docking. I'll call you from Frisco when I land. Oh, my!!

What a frantic year we've spent. How hard we worked is a rich and wonderful memory of wonderful people, brave guys, loyal, caring friends, officers and enlisted men in a wonderful organization.

The last three months have sped by with preparations for Japan, leaving our mother outfit, the 126th, then doing detached services with the 73rd Field, the 116th Station, now here at the 44th General. They didn't want us to get in a rut. No way.

Looking back on this tour of duty, it has been crammed with excitement, hardship, happiness, sorrow, some fleeting depressed times, but over all, these months have flown. I will always be grateful and glad that I got my finger in this pie as I planned when I changed direction from geology to nursing.

It will take me a while to put all this time in perspective. There is much to think about and plan on, but better at home than here ...

Love, Sally B.

November 20, 1945

Dear Mom and Dad,

... Still dreaming of the final word to go home. We know it is coming soon. In the meantime, we are all working very hard. This Officers' Ward is very busy and a lot of fun. We all laugh a lot on duty. Laughter is a great healer. These guys are sharp and educated and fun to be with. So, if I must be here still, it's fun to be here!

When I do get home, I have some requests — a bottle of champagne, two quarts of milk, many blankets and hot water bottles. I'm just sorry all my friends and I will be split up. Nothing like this camaraderie will ever be quite the same again, I know, because the shared dangers, anxieties, exhaustion, gripes, illnesses, fun times, friendships can never be the same. It has been the most wonderful experience of my life, so far.

You both sound so busy and happy with all that is going on in your lives and in your community. It will be an experience to get home to live in a house with all my family, with china on the table. I think I'll remember how to cope.

When we get to the States, we go across country to Fort Dix in New Jersey. I'll be separated there and then have 45 days leave. Won't make Christmas, but I'll love to be home, put on a dress, any dress, just to get rid of these uniform pants! I've worn these shirts and pants so long!

Love, Me

Relieved of Duty — Replacement Depot

November 26, 1945

Dear Mom and Dad,

Yesterday was our day! We were relieved of duty after working all morning. Last night we came down to the Replacement Depot. If we go tonight, we will go on the *Santa Monica*. If we don't, we'll fly to Manila and go from there. Who knows, maybe neither. (*We went on neither plan!*)

It was funny yesterday morning when I woke up, the sky was red and the ocean beautiful. I had a feeling it would be that day and I told Shirl so. The night before, I had washed, starched and ironed all my clothes. For the first time I ever have moved in this man's (and woman's) Army, I am ready! My main problem is that my suitcase is full. I can't believe I've collected so much stuff. Oh, well, I'll leave a lot here.

We're all together again, BC, Betty, Mickey and all the other casuals we came over with. We leave tomorrow!!

Love, Sally B.

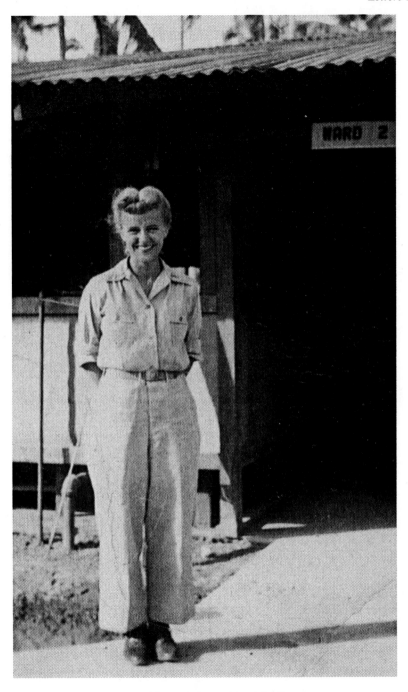

Relieved of duty at noon, November 26, 1945.

CHAPTER SIX

Going Home

At Sea on the *Harry Lee*, Navy APA

December 11, 1945

Dear Mom and Dad,

We have come to Pearl Harbor for minor repairs. Supposedly we will arrive at Dock #7 in Frisco on December 18. We've heard that there is such a bottleneck in Frisco, we may be diverted somewhere else.

We did leave Leyte on November 28 on a Navy APA, the *Harry Lee*. Such quarters we have — four in a room, dressers, mirrors, private showers and a john. It is wonderful. The crew and officers are pleasant. We've had fun aboard, but lately have been on tenterhooks about the water situation. Guess we'll get it fixed at Pearl Harbor.

Love, Sally B.

Delay in Honolulu

December 12, 1945

Dear Mom and Dad,

The officers have asked us to go on shore with them into Honolulu to have a good time. Civilization at last. So we dressed up in our Class A uniforms with all our ribbons and battle stars and overseas stripes and our meritorious awards and went into town. It was a miracle we could wear our uniforms because on shipboard, with GOOD food, and no exercise, we all gained.

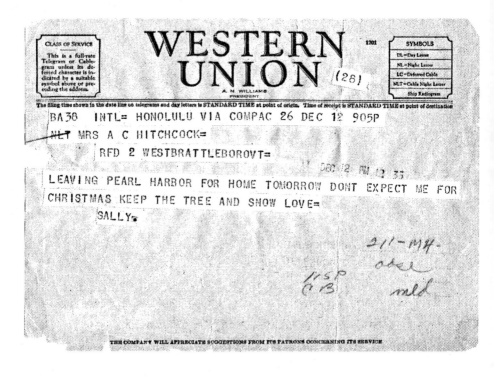

We had a full night in Honolulu, going from hot spot to hot spot, walked on Waikiki, which I found was pretty narrow. I'm not sure it really was Waikiki, but we were told it was. We walked the streets; we danced and came home in the wee hours having been treated to a real night out. The officer who took me was Bill C. He kept referring to the *Harry Lee* as a "bucket of bolts" which would be decommissioned as soon as we hit the States.

We've had a rough trip, pitching and rolling for a week. Chairs, dishes all slid around (the table clothes were wet to keep the dishes on the table). Shirl and I were not sick, but some were.

The rolling was something. Shirl and I almost died laughing one night when all the bottles on our bureau, shampoo, mineral oil and medicine took off like planes and smashed all over the floor. It was hard just standing up against the roll, but with a well-oiled floor it was terrible.

We got a broom from a crew member, then we diluted the oil on the floor with what was left of my precious shampoo and made a ghastly emulsion stirring with the broom. We laughed so hard. This did not help. Then we tried to blot it all up with toilet paper, trying hard not to fall into it each time the ship rolled. It was a tedious task and it took great skill not to sit in it. We won! How the floor shone! I'm sure the Navy was very proud of the job we did. There was a pervading smell of shampoo wafting through the corridors. Trying to sleep against the rolls was a real task. We all won. We learned to sleep.

I shall always remember the chant we hear daily — "Now hear this! Now hear this! Man your brooms! Clean sweep-down fore and aft! Garbage over the fantail!" Never to be forgotten!

Merry Christmas, you three! Save the tree for me. It won't be the lovely palm tree filled with fireflies I saw last year. That was a sight I'll always remember. A real tree will be a thrill and it will smell of balsam!

Have to tell you one other thing. Before we got to Pearl we had a water shortage so, enroute we decided to throw our pants and shirts over the side when they were dirty. But we were called by the captain to his quarters and told not to do that anymore because boats and Army planes seeing Army uniforms would feel a plane or ship had gone down and they would begin a search for survivors. No more heaving of clothes overboard. We now just pack them in the bottom of the suitcase for use at home!! A somewhat different visit to a captain's quarters than we had in Hollandia!! We have learned a lot!

> Much love, Me
> See you soon!!

Stateside — San Diego to Fort Dix
A Private Car and the Trip Home

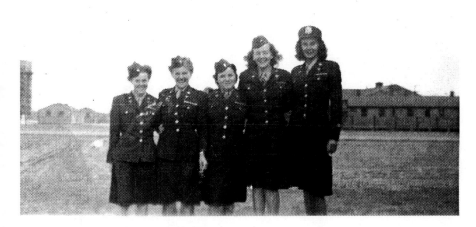

At Camp Anza: Betty, me, Mickey, BC and Shirl.

I remember —

We arrived in San Diego instead of Frisco because of the jammed facilities up north. Much of this landing was a blur. We did land in the USA on the 20th of December. I do remember taking a trolley or electric train into Los Angeles where we went to a telephone company to place our calls home. We left our information for the telephone operators who were swamped with returnees from the Pacific. There were hundreds of us. We were told it would be hours, like four or five or six or more!

So we went to a drugstore to get a glass of milk!! Ice cream!! So good, then we went to the movies. Saw "Lost Weekend" with Ray

Milland. I believe we stopped for a meal. Eventually we went back to the phone company to wait.

The call came through. Our calls were numbered. It was wonderful to talk to my mother, father and brother in Brattleboro, Vermont. It was not yet Christmas, but close. We all knew we'd not make it on time, but here we were in the States.

We met busses that took us up into the hills through orange groves to a place called Camp Anza. We were to wait there for train transport across the country along with thousands of others all waiting. We were there until December 22.

I recall there was an SOS call for the first twelve nurses on orders to get ready to go back to Los Angeles. My name was on that list. I was number 12. We were to be taken to Mr. William Jeffers' (retiring President of Union Pacific R.R.) private car that was to be attached to a troop train as far as Chicago. Was I lucky!

The Los Angeles Herald Express featured a picture of the twelve of us at the tailgate of this private car in the December 22, 1945 edition. The article said:

The Saturday Pictorial Herald Express
Army Nurses
12 in L.A. Agree There Is a Santa

"Tell the folks to keep the Christmas tree up."

"I'm going to sit in a tub and soak for hours — with nobody to tell me to hurry."

These were typical reactions from 12 Army nurses en route today to Fort Dix, New Jersey, in the private car of William M. Jeffers, retiring Union Pacific President, whose gesture to the Army is making the car available to the Leyte returnees to be home for Christmas.

Attached to the Los Angeles Limited, the special car will pull into New York Monday, where the nurses, after spending Christmas with their parents and friends, will report to Fort Dix for separation.

Lieut. Sally Hitchcock's special request is to ski once more, while Lieut. Helen E. Gestwicki wants "oodles and oodles" of fresh vegetables and ice cream. Lieut. Ruth Dailey's Christmas wish lies in a future wedding date with her fiancé still in Leyte.

They all agreed, "There is a Santa Claus."[24]

We didn't travel all the way to New York in that "plushy" car! In Chicago, we were transferred to a troop train bound for Fort Dix.

The trip across to Chicago was unbelievable. We had our own porter and staff, all of whom spoiled us. We ate well, had cocktail

---

[24] The Saturday Pictorial Herald Express, Vol. LXXV, No. 233, December 22, 1945, pg. 1.

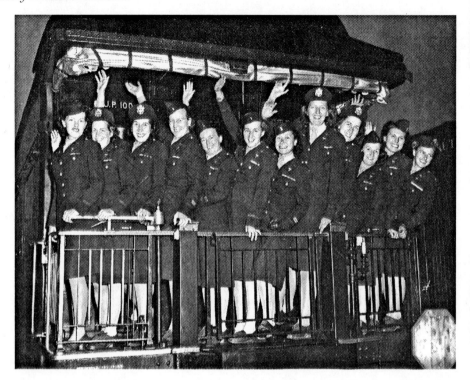

(CA 10) LOS ANGELES, Dec. 21—NURSES RIDE IN JEFFERS' PRIVATE CAR—Twelve Army nurses, who faced the prospect of another Christmas away from home because of the transportation crush, stand on the private railroad car of William Jeffers, president of Union Pacific, who ordered it attached to a Chicago-bound train and offered its use to the Army. Left to right, Sue Allard, Endicott, N.Y.,; Myrtle Ard, Bridgeport, Conn.; Ruth Dailey, Newton Center, Mass.; Dorothy Gage, New Bedford, Mass.; Helen Casey, Wilmington, Del.; Mildred Damon, Bridgeport, Conn.; Ernestine Arnold, N.Y.C.; Rebecca Benedict, Rutland, Vt.; June Bickmore, Manchester, Conn.; Rosemarie Boylan, N.Y.C.; Helen Gestwicki, Dunkirk, N.Y. and Sally Hitchcock, West Brattleboro, Vt. All are 1st Lieutenants. (AP Wirephoto)1945

hour, saw winter scenery. In a little town outside Laramie, Wyoming, three girls got off to buy something and the train left without them. They hired a taxi to drive them at high speed to Laramie where they reboarded. They were lucky!!

Fort Dix, New Jersey

The train ride to Fort Dix from Chicago was uneventful. The countryside was white and cold. We were just like every other soldier on that train who had to be separated at Fort Dix.

But, because of my health history, my separation was delayed. Everyone else left for home. I was admitted to the hospital for "TESTS." Again, I went through the old routine. After three days, I was sent on my way home.

Home

Armed with all my papers, suitcase (no pail anymore and I'm sorry I didn't bring it home, it was such a friend) and my joy, I got on the train, hit the New York, New Haven and Hartford line up the coast to New Haven; then up the familiar Connecticut Valley, through Meriden, Berlin, Hartford, Windsor in Connecticut, then to Springfield, Northampton and Greenfield in Massachusetts (where I had left from in June, 1944) and eventually to Brattleboro, Vermont.

On the platform, waiting, were my family, Mom, Dad and brother John. I was home! What an emotional moment!

When I went through the front door of the house, all the lights were on. The tree was aglow and the long-dreamt-of scent of Christmas balsam greeted me. It was a joyous moment. We were all there, safe and sound, together. The war was finally, truly over. I never shall forget.

After 45 days of terminal leave, I was honorably discharged from the Army on February 15, 1946 and a new chapter of my life began.

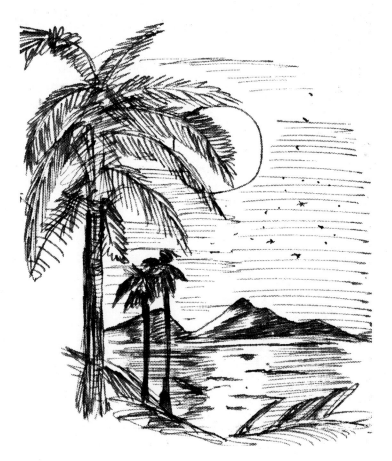

A memory

Epilogue

All of this happened a long time ago. It was a terrible time, an inspiring time, a sad and wonderful time, a time which molded all of us into people different from the persons we had been before.

When the war ended, life went on. Many of the deep friendships we formed then have continued to the present. BC, Shirl and I were all happily married and had families. Now all of us have grandchildren and are widowed. Mickey and Betty never married and are now gone.

Shirl and I made real careers of nursing. Shirl was skilled in school nursing and I worked in several areas of nursing, including public health, as a nursing school instructor, a supervisor and finally as a geriatric nurse practitioner. BC furthered her education and has tutored for many years.

ER and Dan each married, had families, went to school and made the Army their careers. After retirement, each taught in a second career.

Sadly, I have lost track of many wonderful Army friends. The good side for me is that the memory of these friends is frozen in time. Their faces remain forever young, their bodies straight and slim, and their smiles bright.

Pictures in my album, although faded and yellow, recall so much. Looking at the pictures and reading the letters I wrote to my parents and friends renewed for me this period vividly, and sometimes painfully, as I wrote down my memories.

Now there is a sense of deep relief that I am able to put away my big box of letters. The main events are written down on paper. The forging of deep friendships was real and has lasted all these years. I am blessed. I hope you have enjoyed sharing with the person-I-was and my good friends as we experienced this turbulent time and helped in this great endeavor.

PAX VOBISCUM
(Peace be with you)

ABOUT THE AUTHOR

The author, now an octogenarian, looks at her long life as full, varied and exciting. A graduate of Smith College, 1941, and Yale University School of Nursing, 1944, she joined the Army Nurse Corps immediately following graduation and spent the next two years in military service in New Guinea and the Philippines. She worked as head nurse in the Newington Veterans Hospital in Connecticut until she married in 1948. The next years were spent raising three children, with community activities, teaching nursing, providing visiting nurse services, gardening, travelling, and rehabilitating an old Vermont farm.

Now a widow, the author lives in the same 250 year old house the family moved to 44 years ago. She loves mowing her lawn and raising and selling raspberries. She tends her flowers, enjoys the piano and listening to tapes of the oldies from the 30's and 40's. She still drives to see family in Vermont and Pennsylvania and flies to Texas to see her eldest. She serves on the library board and in her church. She proof reads and writes for the local monthly newspaper. Her newest challenge is e-mail to keep in touch with many friends and children and grandchildren. She is actively engaged in environmental causes and political activities. Each day continues to be too short.

Printed in the United States
23735LVS00005B/43-51

9 781418 427894